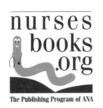

The Publishing Program of ANA

FAITH COMMUNITY NURSING:

DEVELOPING A QUALITY PRACTICE

CAROL J. SMUCKER, PHD, RN

LINDA WEINBERG, PHD, RN, NP, ET
CONTRIBUTING AUTHOR

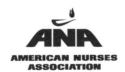

American Nurses Association
Silver Spring, Maryland
2009

Library of Congress Cataloging-in-Publication Data

Smucker, Carol J.
  Faith community nursing : developing a quality practice / Carol J. Smucker
with Linda Weinberg, contributing author.
      p. ; cm.
  Includes bibliographical references and index.
  ISBN-13: 978-1-55810-252-1 (pbk.)
  ISBN-10: 1-55810-252-3 (pbk.)
  1. Parish nursing. 2. Community health nursing. 3. Spirituality. I. Weinberg, Linda.
II. American Nurses Association. III. Title.
[DNLM: 1. Community Health Nursing. 2. Spirituality. 3. Holistic Nursing.
 4. Quality Assurance, Health Care. WY 87 S666f 2008]

  RT120.P37S68 2008
  610.73'43—dc22   2008028359

The opinions in this book reflect those of the authors and do not necessarily reflect positions or policies of the American Nurses Association. Furthermore, the information in this book should not be construed as legal or other professional advice.

Published by Nursesbooks.org
The Publishing Program of ANA

American Nurses Association
8515 Georgia Avenue, Suite 400
Silver Spring, MD 20910-3492
1-800-274-4ANA
www.Nursesbooks.org

ANA is the only full-service professional organization representing the nation's 2.9 million Registered Nurses through its 54 constituent member associations. ANA advances the nursing profession by fostering high standards of nursing practice, promoting the economic and general welfare of nurses in the workplace, projecting a positive and realistic view of nursing, and lobbying the Congress and regulatory agencies on healthcare issues affecting nurses and the public.

Page and cover design: Stacy Maguire, Eyedea Advertising and Design, Sterling, VA

Development editing: Rosanne O'Connor Roe, ANA ~ *Production editing:* Eric Wurzbacher, ANA

Copyediting: Lisa Munsat Anthony, Chapel Hill, NC ~ *Indexing:* Estalita Slivoskey, Ellendale, ND

Proofreading: Ashley Mason, Jackson Heights, NY ~ *Printing:* McArdle Printing, Upper Marlboro, MD

Compostion: Stacy Maguire, Eyedea Advertising and Design, Sterling, VA

ISBN-13: 978-1-55810-252-1   SAN: 851-3481   2.5M   11/08

First printing November 2008.

CONTENTS

Transitioning to the Faith Community Nursing (FCN) role often involves moving from a high-tech to a low-tech environment. Faith community nursing emphasizes *being with* people rather than *doing for* them. An FCN (Faith Community Nurse) needs to understand this ministry of presence to successfully establish a health ministry in a faith community. This chapter highlights the elements of spiritual nursing care and ways to develop spiritual care skills. Helpful suggestions are provided as the nurse begins work in the faith community setting.

Nurses begin work in a faith community knowing what it is like to be a faith community member. Being a part of the staff requires the FCN to see the faith community, its staff, and one's self from a different perspective. Each FCN will experience an adjustment period related to his or her prior expectations. This chapter encourages the FCN to be inquisitive and open to new ways of doing things. Suggestions are given for ensuring that the FCN's relationships within the faith community and the surrounding community are effective from the beginning to avoid future problems. The FCN, with a well-established health ministry, often plays a key role during change in faith community leadership.

The overall purpose of faith community nursing is to help a faith community understand the interrelationship between faith and health and help people live this relationship out to achieve whole-person health. The FCN follows the nursing process, adapting it to the faith community setting. Faith community nursing requires the nurse to be knowledgeable of religious, health, and community resources in order to serve as a link between these and the faith community's health needs.

This chapter emphasizes the importance of professional practice. It gives time-conscious ways to meet the accountability expectations of the faith community, healthcare system, and nursing standards.

An important part of the FCN role is working with volunteers—getting others involved in the health ministry. This involves recruiting, training, and recognizing those who help. An immediate source of volunteers will be your Health Committee members. Sharing the work with others will not only build a solid foundation for your work, but keep you from feeling as though you have to do it all yourself.

Drawing a picture of a healthy tree and discussing analogies for wholistic health are fun educational exercises. This chapter applies the metaphor of a healthy tree for the ongoing health of the FCN. The FCN is encouraged to take care of mind, body, and spirit in order to have the *well-being* to continually draw from in order to care for and comfort others.

This chapter will explain the model of Jewish congregational nursing to both those who will practice in a synagogue or Jewish community setting and faith-based nurses who are interested in expanding their knowledge base. The model of Jewish Congregational Nursing is based upon Jewish history, philosophy, texts, and religious practices that have common ground among Orthodox, Conservative, Reform, and Reconstructive branches of the Jewish religion. Jewish nurses from all backgrounds will be able to use this model to practically set up programs in their respective settings.

As faith community nursing moves into the twenty-first century, it continues to evolve. Some basic practice issues continue to be debated and new issues emerge to challenge FCNs to address them in constructive and creative ways.

ACKNOWLEDGMENTS

Many thanks to my husband, David, and family and friends who continue to encourage my writing. With appreciation to faith community nurse contributors Judy Glancy, Rachel Hallam, Carol Hamilton, Jackie Herzlinger, Vonda Jennings, Barbara Marlin, Michelle Pearce, Lisa Sinclair, Carol Tippe, and Linda Weinberg for their wisdom. Thanks to my good friend, Judy Barnette, for allowing me to tell her story. With gratitude to Rosanne O'Connor Roe, my editor, for giving me the opportunity to write this book and always challenging me to say it better.

And for their invaluable insights and suggestions, I thank my reviewers, many of whom are dear friends and faith community nursing colleagues: Sharon Adkins, Joan Bard, Carol Bickford, Nancy Durbin, Janet Griffin, Lisa Sinclair, Mary Slutz, Sharon Stanton, Wendy Stiver, and Lisa Zerull. Special thanks to Rev. David Carlson and all the chaplains I've worked with who taught me about spiritual care.

Carol Smucker, PhD, RN

With extreme thanks to my late husband Marc, my children, friends, and family who both encouraged and showed great patience toward me in my academic and professional career. Thanks to Libby Blackman, Jean Redstone, and Janna Dieckman for their valuable insights. For his wisdom and steadiness, Eduard vanHulst. Much appreciation to Rosanne O'Connor Roe for giving me the opportunity to share with others thoughts about Jewish Congregational Nursing. Gratitude to Rabbi David Mayer, Leah and Bill Margolis, and Morris and Joyce Shor, who continues to teach me about how to live one's life in a Jewish tradition.

Linda Weinberg, PhD, RN, NP, ET

ABOUT THE AUTHORS

Carol J. Smucker, PhD, RN, is the former Parish Nurse Program Coordinator for Baptist Hospital of East Tennessee, Knoxville, Tennessee. She is co-author of the book *Nursing the Spirit* (Wilt and Smucker 2001). She worked in acute care settings and taught nursing at Lutheran Hospital School for Nurses, Moline, Illinois; University of Iowa; and the University of Tennessee-Knoxville. She has presented her research at national conferences and is published in nursing journals and books. Her doctoral research was on spiritual distress. She completed the Health Ministry Education program at Lutheran Hospital, Des Moines, Iowa, and served as parish nurse for Zion Lutheran Church, Davenport, Iowa.

Linda Weinberg, PhD, RN, NP, ET, has a background as both a family nurse practitioner and Jewish para-chaplain, served as a Jewish Congregational Nurse through Philadelphia Jewish Family and Children's service and her synagogue in Phoenixville, PA. She taught community health nursing at the University of Pennsylvania and Allentown College. She has presented her research at various national conferences. Her doctoral dissertation was concerned with the clinical thinking of undergraduate nursing students. She also has an expertise in dermatology and wound care.

INTRODUCTION

FAITH COMMUNITY NURSES are now so widely distributed in the United States, you are likely to encounter them wherever you go. In 2005 I was in Orlando, Florida, taking part in a Stephen Ministry Leadership Training Conference. Following one learning activity, the person I was working with became my prayer partner for the week. In talking with my prayer partner, I discovered we were both nurses and, surprisingly, also had experience as faith community nurses (FCNs), she in Pennsylvania and I in Iowa.

Another discovery of mutual interest in faith community nursing occurred at a dinner in my North Carolina church. I sat next to a woman who was visiting family in our area. As we got acquainted, I learned about her work as an FCN in Iowa. These are just two recent examples of the many FCNs I have met recently in traveling around the country.

Although no one knows the exact number of FCNs worldwide, it is estimated to be about 8,000. Rev. Granger Westberg, faith community nursing's founder (then called parish nursing), would be amazed. Look up this relatively new nursing specialty on the Internet today and you'll find thousands of sites listed. These include faith community nursing education programs, regional FCN programs, the International Parish Nurse Resource Center, the Health Ministries Association, faith communities with an FCN on staff, and even FCNs' individual Web sites. In the two decades since faith community nursing began in the Chicago area in 1984, it has spread across the United States and to other countries (for example, the United Kingdom, Canada, Australia, New Zealand, South Africa, Swaziland, and Korea).

FCNs around the world are leaders in this innovative nursing practice within faith-based settings. Faith community nursing promotes wholistic health through intentional care of the spirit, health promotion, disease prevention, and disease management strategies, drawing on the resources of each person's religious belief system. The FCN helps people understand the interrelationship of faith and health which empowers and enriches life. FCNs work in both paid and unpaid positions. Some FCNs are employees of hospital systems or health agencies while others are hired directly by faith communities.

This handbook provides basic information for the beginning FCN. It addresses liability and other practice concerns of faith community nursing. Faith community nursing standards of practice and professional performance are highlighted and suggested resources listed for each chapter. This book is not intended to be a faith community nursing textbook or a substitute for a formal faith community nursing education program. Many excellent texts and programs exist to provide the necessary knowledge base for faith community nursing practice. However, what has not been available is information about the reality of working as a nurse in a faith community and the challenge of creating and shaping a type of nursing practice that is still new and largely unknown to the public. This book describes the experiences of two faith community nurses and, in doing so, it attempts to show those nurses new to the specialty examples of practice procedures. These examples are not intended to be viewed as the only possible approaches to FCN.

My faith community nursing experience began with the Health Minister Education Program at Iowa Lutheran Hospital, Des Moines, Iowa, in 1986–87, combined with serving as an FCN in a Lutheran church in Davenport, Iowa. In 1994 in Knoxville, Tennessee, I helped start one of the state's first faith community nursing programs through Baptist Hospital and served as Coordinator for six years. Thus, this book is a result of much early trial and error as one of the first FCNs in the United States and my experience as an FCN program developer and coordinator. I have contributed to faith community nursing's development by participating in curriculum development work with the International Parish Nurse Resource Center, presenting at the Westberg Symposium, and as a member of the Southeast Coordinator's Group.

Although my experience in faith community nursing is with Christian faith communities, this book is based on *Faith Community Nursing: Scope and Standards of Practice*, co-published by the American Nurses Association and the Health Ministries Association, and should be useful to most FCNs working in other faith communities.

I am grateful for Linda Weinberg's contribution of a chapter on her model of Jewish Congregational Nursing and Jackie Herzlinger's contributions on her work in Jewish faith communities.

For each chapter, I've pulled out the main practice principles and highlighted them for a quick reference. Although faith community nursing practice will continue to evolve, these guiding principles should remain helpful for years to come.

I have learned about faith community nursing and spiritual care from many people. Although it is not possible to name them all here, I want to recognize Chaplain David Carlson, who started the Health Minister Education Program in Iowa and was co-founder of the Health Ministries Association. I learned much from his excellent leadership and teaching, especially in the area of spiritual care.

During the last class day in my Health Minister Education Program, Chaplain Carlson asked the class to write down fears about starting to practice in what is now called faith community nursing. One of my concerns was whether faith communities would value this type of ministry and how long it would last. Although it is still a struggle for faith communities to reimburse FCNs, there is no doubt, from the sheer number of nurses practicing faith community nursing, that it *is* valued and meeting many healthcare needs. Faith community nursing practice continues to spread across this country and around the world. It appears that faith community nursing is only now at the beginning of what it will be in the future.

I wrote this book because I value faith community nursing and enjoy teaching nurses. It has been rewarding to work with a variety of FCNs and faith communities to help establish and develop successful faith community nursing practices.

All of you reading this book are a part of the future of a faith community nursing. I hope you are committed to helping faith community nursing continue to grow and develop. I trust this book will be a helpful companion to you on your faith community nursing journey. My prayers are with you. I know your journey will be an amazing one, and I'm glad to be a part of it through this book.

Carol J. Smucker, PhD, RN
Brasstown, North Carolina
October 2007

CHAPTER 1

FAITH COMMUNITY NURSING: DEVELOPMENT OF STANDARDS

Faith community nursing is the specialized practice of professional nursing that focuses on the intentional care of the spirit as part of the process of promoting wholistic health and preventing or minimizing illness in a faith community.

The goal of the faith community nurse (FCN) is the protection, promotion, and optimization of health and abilities; prevention of illness and injury; and responding to suffering in the context of the values, beliefs, and practices of a faith community such as a church, congregation, parish, synagogue, temple, or mosque (ANA and HMA 2005, p. 1).

FROM THE TIME faith community nursing began in the 1980s as parish nursing, many of its leaders saw the need for specialty nursing standards. Parish nurse education programs were developing in different parts of the country, but many nurses were starting to work in faith communities on their own with little guidance or direction. Beginning in 1987, parish nurses and others interested in learning more about parish nursing met together in the Chicago area for what became an annual conference sponsored by the International Parish Nurse Resource Center (IPNRC). This conference, now held in St. Louis, Missouri, continues to provide opportunities for networking, worship, and continuing education.

The IPNRC's mission is to promote the development of quality parish nurse programs through research, education, and consultation. In this regard, the IPNRC regularly surveyed parish nurses and parish nurse coordinators to determine parish nursing's scope of practice. With the IPNRC's support and guidance, parish nursing began to spread rapidly throughout the country.

It became clear to some parish nurses that common standards would help parish nurses develop quality practices and hasten recognition of this nursing specialty as a significant addition to community health

> Whatever their educational background, all faith community nurses have a common focus: the intentional care of the spirit. This is what makes faith community nursing unique.

care. The Health Ministries Association, Inc. (HMA) was started to serve a global multi-faith membership interested in developing whole-person ministries in faith communities and the communities they serve. It became the professional membership organization for parish nurses and took the leadership in developing parish nursing standards. *Scope and Standards of Parish Nursing Practice* was published jointly by HMA and the American Nurses Association (ANA) in 1998 and revised and retitled in 2005 as *Faith Community Nursing: Scope and Standards of Practice*.

The first *Standards of Nursing Practice* was published by ANA in 1973. As nursing specialties proliferated, their standards have also been published. Revisions of the original standards have followed, with the current *Nursing: Scope and Standards of Practice* being published in 2004. With this publication, as well as the publication of *Nursing's Social Policy Statement* (ANA 2003) and *Code of Ethics for Nurses with Interpretive Statements* (ANA 2001), all specialty scope and standards are being revised, modeled on the 2004 standards.

Nursing standards describe and guide the development of nursing practice. They provide a document that communicates nursing's values and responsibilities to the public, healthcare organizations, and other professionals. They delineate the nursing profession and provide a means for accountability and evaluation. They describe a competent level of nursing care. The ultimate purpose of nursing standards, of course, is to improve the health and quality of life of people receiving nursing care.

While the 2004 scope and standards publication provides a broad framework for nursing practice, the comparable publication for faith community nursing incorporates specialty terminology (such as *faith community* and *spiritual leader*) and describes the unique scope of knowledge, standards of care, and professional performance expected of an FCN (ANA and HMA 2005). All FCNs should refer to the FCN standards to answer questions about the *who, what, where, when, why,* and *how* of FCN practice. Nursing standards are dynamic and expected to change as FCNs test them in practice and knowledge and as technology and healthcare systems continue to evolve.

Included in the revised standards are measurement criteria for advanced practice registered nurses (nurse practitioners, certified registered nurse anesthetists, certified nurse midwives, and clinical nurse specialists). These criteria describe additional responsibilities expected from these specialists. The education of the advanced practice registered nurses enables them to care for complex patients and health situations and be leaders in the nursing profession. Lisa Sinclair, an APRN, speaks to this perspective:

I manage our program of paid parish nurses and unpaid congregational health promoters (CHPs). As an APRN Family Nurse Practitioner, I find that I am able to provide a different world view. I am able to help the nurses and CHPs locate their particular congregation in the greater context of community epidemiology, health disparities, U.S. health trends, and world need. Additionally, I am able to provide the framework of nursing skills competency. I know the training that is needed to grow in and maintain clinical excellence. Because I have another master's [degree] from seminary, I am able to help bridge the gap between the normal nursing scope and the pastoral care function of the FCN. Accordingly, I see a big role for APRNs in the leadership and practice of our specialty.

Whether the advanced practice registered nurse, FCN, fully uses all legally allowed interventions, such as prescriptive authority, depends on the needs and desires of the faith community in which that nurse works. Whatever their educational background, all faith community nurses have a common focus: the intentional care of the spirit. This is what makes faith community nursing unique.

All faith community nursing standards are incorporated in the chapters ahead. Practice examples are provided which show practical ways the standards can be put into practice. I encourage you to read this book with the standards in hand. As you practice, consult your standards frequently, communicate them to the faith community, discuss them with colleagues, and challenge each other to put them into practice. Regularly read through them and evaluate your practice in relationship to them. Practicing by these standards will help you develop and maintain a quality practice.

REFERENCES AND RESOURCES

All online references and resources were current September 30, 2008.

REFERENCES

American Nurses Association (ANA) and Health Ministries Association (HMA). 2005. *Faith community nursing: Scope and standards of practice.* Silver Spring, MD: Nursesbooks.org.

SUGGESTED RESOURCES

American Nurses Association (ANA). 2001. *Code of ethics for nurses with interpretive statements.* Washington, DC: American Nurses Association.

_____. 2003. *Nursing's social policy statement,* 2nd ed. Silver Spring, MD: Nursesbooks.org.

_____. 2004. *Nursing: Scope and standards of practice.* Silver Spring, MD: Nursesbooks.org.

ORGANIZATIONAL RESOURCES

Health Ministries Association Web site: **www.hmassoc.org**

International Parish Nurse Resource Center Web site: **www.ipnrc.parishnurses.org**

CHAPTER 2

BEING AND DOING: THE FCN ROLE TRANSITION

During a discussion about hiring a faith community nurse (FCN), a faith community member asks, "Why do we need a nurse? It's not often that someone falls down and hurts themselves here."

PEOPLE ARE NATURALLY CONFUSED by faith community nursing. When most people think of nurses, they think of the nurse in their doctor's office or the one who cared for them in the hospital. They usually picture a nurse giving physical care and find it difficult to transfer this image to the faith community. Then when they learn that FCNs do not usually give this type of care, they are doubly confused. What then, they ask, will the nurse do? Spoken or unspoken, the question "Why do we need a nurse?" is present in every faith community that has a nurse on staff. You will want to address this question, especially at the beginning of your ministry, to help the faith community understand your role and periodically thereafter to refresh memories and inform new members.

INTRODUCING FAITH COMMUNITY NURSING AND WHOLISTIC HEALTH

For many nurses, practicing in a faith community seems a natural extension of their nursing role. In fact, they sometimes feel as though they're working when faith community friends come up to them and ask health questions. But having a nurse on the staff is a new and somewhat strange idea to most faith communities. To my knowledge, it is only some of the African-American faith communities which have traditionally had a group of women called *nurses* assisting members during worship services. Most faith communities have not had formal roles or staff positions for professional nurses.

In talking to many different faith communities about faith community nursing, I came to realize that part of the confusion over the role is because many people do not fully understand nursing practice itself, especially how broadly a nurse is educated. This is not surprising, since few nurses are able to practice their profession fully in most healthcare settings. Thus, when you begin, you have a wonderful opportunity to educate people about nurses: their role in promoting wholistic health and preventing or minimizing illness. (*Wholistic*: the *w* was added to holism by Rev. Granger Westberg to emphasize the theological concept of wholeness or unity of the mind, body, and spirit. Wholism is an accepted and important concept to nurses who consider the whole person greater than its parts.)

One way to help your faith community and its spiritual leaders understand the FCN role is to introduce *Faith Community Nursing: Scope and Standards of Practice* to them. A lot of good discussion will be stimulated by explaining the FCN's goal: *to protect, promote, and optimize health and abilities, prevent illness and injury, and respond to suffering in the context of the values, beliefs, and practices of a faith community* (ANA and HMA 2005, p. 1). You can include in your discussion the current popular interest in the relationship between faith and health as well as complementary health care, which includes spiritual interventions, such as meditation. Explore with them their own and their faith community's beliefs about health and healing. They'll also be interested to learn of the historic role faith communities have played in promoting health and healing and how faith community nursing is helping them reclaim that role today. Questions you might ask are: "In what ways should the faith community be responsible for the health of its members?" and "How does faith impact health, and vice versa?"

Talking about the faith community's role in health and healing will be a natural lead-in to tell about faith community nursing's theological roots and its development as parish nursing in the 1980s with Rev. Granger Westberg. Faith community nursing's focus on health and healing is rooted in Judeo-Christian traditions which reflect a Hebrew, or Old Testament, understanding of health in which the physical and spiritual aspects of health and healing are inseparable. It is also modeled on a New Testament understanding of Jesus' ministry of teaching, preaching, and healing—addressing the concerns of mind, body, and spirit wholistically. For example, Christ's physical healings often included spiritual healings. Although faith community nursing attributes these beliefs to its beginning within the Christian community, other faiths also hold similar beliefs about health and healing. Within the faith group where you practice, build your discussion about health on that group's belief system.

As you help people understand the interrelationship between the physical, emotional, and spiritual aspects of their lives, you'll assist people to practice good spiritual habits as well as good physical and mental ones. This will enable people to work toward a healthy mind–body–spirit balance. Because most people associate good health primarily with physical health, it is easy to neglect mental and spiritual health. We can even lose sight of the larger purpose for being healthy. For people of faith, health is never an end in itself, but rather a means to living out that faith in the world.

Communicating and explaining your role to the faith community will continue throughout your ministry because some people will always be unfamiliar with it. Over time, more people will understand better what you do as word spreads about your role. You'll be surprised that even those people who were initially opposed to having an FCN often change their minds and become the FCN's greatest proponents when they or someone they know is helped by the FCN.

Wholistic Health

Most people are familiar with the term *holistic*. You can expand on this understanding as you explain the reason faith community nursing uses the spelling *wholistic* to emphasize the concept of wholeness or whole-person health. Some of the main ideas about wholistic health that you'll want to communicate are:

- A person cannot be truly healthy without a healthy spirit. The spirit is both a part of our essential human nature and transcends the physical. It is concerned with meaning, faith, hope, love, peace, and healthy relationships with self, others, the environment, and the divine.

- Spiritual health can be a powerful resource for recovering from illness and maintaining good overall health.

- Even in chronic illness or impending death, times when the physical body and mind are diminishing, persons of faith can experience health as a sense of well-being because of the spiritual peace, courage, and strength that enables them to manage their condition and live as fully as possible under the circumstances.

- Spiritual health and physical health are inseparable aspects of the person and constantly interacting.

- A person can be physically well, but spiritually sick.

- Spiritual concerns over time can negatively affect physical, emotional, and mental well-being.

- Healing is not only physical. It can involve emotional and mental healing as well as healing of memories and relationships.

BEGINNING WORK: GETTING ACQUAINTED AND SPREADING THE WORD

Getting to know people and becomming known are critical to faith community nursing, as it is a ministry accomplished through relationships. Whether you're working in a small rural faith community or with a large urban congregation, you'll seek out opportunities to get acquainted with the whole faith community. Wearing a name tag that includes your title makes it easier for people to identify you. You may also want to have business cards that include your contact information to hand out to people. These cards can serve more than one purpose by having a blood pressure record printed on the back of the card for people to use.

A good way to begin to get acquainted is to plan some meetings to talk with the faith community about your role. It's always a good idea to also plan a get-together with the other health professionals in the faith community so they'll be informed about what you're doing and learn ways they can be a part of the health ministry. Although you can't attend every activity on the calendar, select different ones each week to attend to get acquainted. Don't forget to meet and get to know the support staff, such as the administrative assistants and the custodians. You'll be working with them, too, and wanting them to know how what they do contributes to the success of this new ministry. You can also learn a lot from them about how the faith community functions. The first few weeks and months are critical to being accepted. First impressions are important. A smile, a handshake, attentive listening, and caring words will convey friendship and start off your relationship-building right.

Be visible. Think of all the ways you can let people know about your work. Acquire some bulletin board space for providing information about your activities. Why not post a picture of yourself so people can easily identify you? Design a brochure describing faith community nursing and your proposed ministry and activities. Distribute it to various groups in the faith community and leave it in key traffic locations in the faith community building. Attempt to reach all age groups. Take advantage of every opportunity to describe what you do at various faith community meetings. Offer to write a column in the faith community's newsletter or do a special introductory mailing to the congregation. If the faith community has a website, submit information about your ministry and mission, the activities you are planning, and any regular services you provide, such as monthly blood pressure checks.

You may be the first FCN in town! You will be seen as news, and the local media may be interested in doing a story about you and your work. Don't hesitate to appear on radio or TV talk shows or be interviewed for newspapers. And don't forget about your larger faith organization's magazines and newspapers. After you've practiced awhile, you'll have some great success stories to write up for publication. Consider writing an article about your work for a nursing journal. If this seems daunting, find a colleague or nursing professor who has already been published to help you write an article or work with you on a joint article. Faith community nurses have much to contribute to people's understanding of the role of faith in health. I encourage you to tell your stories about the ways you help people through faith community nursing.

An excellent and very meaningful way to initiate your ministry and make it known to the faith community is through an installation or commissioning service. If the faith community does not have one of its own, sample installation services are available through the International Parish Nurse Resource Center (IPNRC).

Faith communities vary as to how quickly they will understand the purpose of faith community nursing. While each faith community usually has a long history of providing health and healing ministry activities for both their own members as well as their surrounding community, they may not be recognized by these terms. Thus, the FCN will help the faith community recognize that the FCN activities will build on and extend this existing health ministry. One of the ways you will broaden and strengthen the existing ministry is by helping to connect people to meet each other's needs, both within the church and as outreach to the larger community.

THE HEALTH COMMITTEE

Forming a health committee within the faith community to support the FCN ministry is recommended by Rev. Granger Westberg as essential to its success. Whether the faith community chooses to call it the Health Committee, the Health Cabinet, or the Health Council, it is a group that is invaluable to beginning and maintaining a quality faith community nursing ministry. If you are a part of a hospital faith community nursing program, the program coordinator may have already worked with the faith community to choose people to develop and serve this group. If not, meet with the faith community spiritual leader to identify people who might have an interest in health ministry and who represent different faith community groups and ages. The committee should be representative of the congregation to help you reach diverse groups and give a broad ownership to the ministry. Some, but not all, should be health professionals. A group of 10 to 12 people works well. When formed, the group should choose a chairperson and a secretary. You, the spiritual leader, and other staff members will be ex officio (non-voting) members.

The health committee should meet regularly, preferably once a month for the first year, until the health ministry is well established. Some faith communities do not have a committee structure but form work groups as the need arises. In that case, I recommend that you find a small group of interested people to meet with you several times a year to get feedback and ideas, and to identify people to help you with projects, especially if you're not serving in your own faith community.

The first meeting of the Health Committee is a good time to get acquainted and to talk about faith community nursing and the ideas you have for the health ministry. (Sometimes the Health Committee has already met you, because they served as the Interview Committee.) Then, the whole group can spend time brainstorming, prioritizing, and generating ideas and decide on a few areas that they see as the faith community's most immediate health needs. Some committee members may want to help you put together the congregational survey (to gather information about the faith community's health needs and interests) and work with you to distribute it and tabulate results. At each meeting you'll provide a monthly report of your work and involve the group in planning for the future.

Although I would recommend retaining a separate health committee, it may work well for you to be a part of an existing committee or group (whose mission is similar to faith community nursing) after you have been at the faith community awhile. Encourage your committee not only to plan with you but to work with you on projects. Judy Glancy, FCN, does this in a large Catholic faith community:

> Our Wellness Committee consists of 12 healthcare professionals, and we offer various programs of interest for parishioners to maintain wellness. Those on the Wellness Committee are also supportive in many other ways, such as taking blood pressures after Masses. They are presently bringing items for a Wellness basket for our basket raffle. It is going to be wonderful!

Choosing people who understand this mission of the faith community and are enthusiastic or knowledgeable about health or healing will create a pool of willing volunteers and encourage others to get involved.

THINGS TO INCLUDE IN A FAITH COMMUNITY HEALTH INTEREST SURVEY

- Your name, title, and contact information
- Reason for the survey
- List of possible health education topics (from which people select topics of interest)
- Space for respondents to write their own health concerns or topics
- Space for respondents to indicate age and gender
- Space for respondents to identify preferred time and day of week for class

THE SCOPE OF FAITH COMMUNITY NURSING PRACTICE

The scope of faith community nursing practice is included in the FCN Standards (ANA and HMA 2005, p. 1). The scope of practice includes the definition and overview of faith community nursing, its evolution, assumptions, and spiritual care focus as well as educational preparation and professional trends and issues. Although the preferred minimum preparation for faith community nursing is a baccalaureate or higher degree in nursing, practicing faith community nurses come from a variety of educational programs.

Faith community nursing practice extends beyond the faith community into the larger community. The health risks for the larger community are also health risks for the faith communities within it. It is important to understand these risks in order to prevent illness and promote health. Other community health concepts such as community health assessment, cultural diversity, and aggregate care are used in faith community nursing (Speck 2003). Therefore, it is important for the FCN to have academic preparation in community health nursing. If this was not a part of your nursing education, find a way to educate yourself in this important component of faith community nursing.

Not only do you need to learn about the larger community's health risks but also its healthcare assets. One of the FCN's main activities is to help people access the most appropriate community resources. To learn more about these, visit key community agencies, such as the health department, the area agency for aging, and hospice services. Also make contact with mental health agencies or professionals in the larger community. After several months of doing this, I had contacted over 20 agencies and gathered a wealth of information. These contacts also provide an opportunity to introduce yourself as a faith community nurse and talk about your role in community health. You may already be familiar with your community's agencies, but if not, taking time to get acquainted will not only give you the information you need to refer people to services, but also begin building good working relationships between you and them.

While faith community nursing is a specialty practice area within nursing because of its intentional focus on spiritual care, the FCN's broad range of activities reflects the generalist nature of faith community nursing. Since most nurses, prior to beginning faith community nursing, will have practiced in a variety of other nursing specialty areas, such as cardiac, respiratory, or mental health, keeping current on a wider variety of health conditions and treatments will be a challenge. I started working as a faith community nurse after a nursing master's program, during which I was not employed as a nurse. Therefore, to provide the most accurate up-to-date health information to people, I read nursing journals, attended professional workshops, and gathered health-related brochures for heart disease, cancer, and other major health conditions to give to people.

Even with your best efforts at continuing learning, there is no way you will have all the knowledge you need to answer every health question people ask you. The most truthful and best response when you don't know the answer is to say "I don't know, but I'll try to find out for you." People will appreciate your honesty and your willingness to search for the information. FCNs who have computer access have a wealth of reliable information at their fingertips and find many reliable health resources for people this way. Nurses can also help people interpret and evaluate health information they find themselves on the Web.

Know your scope of practice as an FCN. Make a realistic assessment of your areas of expertise and knowledge you need to gain to practice according to the FCN Standards. One of your professional responsibilities is to continue learning. Another key learning area for an FCN is that of providing spiritual care. This is an area most nurses will not have been prepared for in their basic nursing program, but it is one the FCN will need to prepare for to fulfill the primary responsibility of faith community nursing: the intentional care of the spirit.

INTENTIONAL CARE OF THE SPIRIT

What is the spirit? The spirit is that part of humans that connects them to the divine or whatever they conceive as the ultimate reality. Many faiths believe that the human spirit lives on after physical death. It is the part of the person that seeks meaning and purpose in life, love, forgiveness, hope, peace, and belief and trust in a transcendent power, energy, or person. Caring for the spirit, then, is assisting people to connect to the transcendent, to feel loved, forgiven, to have hope, and live a meaningful and purposeful life. The FCN provides spiritual care in many ways. Treating people with respect and protecting their dignity is giving spiritual care. Listening to people and helping them express their feelings is spiritual care. Showing compassion and helping alleviate suffering is spiritual care. Basically, spiritual care is helping people to realize wholeness in all aspects of their lives (Sawatzky and Pesut 2005). Spiritual care may be talking with people about their faith and praying with them. More frequently shown, though, spiritual care will simply be the way you relate to people every day in your work: showing them compassion and concern.

Most nurses come to faith community nursing well prepared to be health educators, health counselors, support group leaders, patient advocates, and group facilitators. They easily develop health programs, teach health topics, answer health questions, and guide people to appropriate resources. From my experience hiring nurses for FCN positions, some nurses (who know little about the specialty) think the job is nothing more than doing these things in a church setting. However, for other nurses (who do know about faith community nursing), it is often the spiritual component and being able to speak freely about their faith which attracts them to it. These nurses have always wanted to combine their faith with nursing but have often been unable to do so, at least openly, in their work settings.

Nurses begin faith community nursing at different levels of spiritual experience and maturity. Some may have a seminary degree or have taken spiritual formation courses. Others have a lifelong faith community experience with extensive knowledge of their faith and how to communicate it. Some may be new to their faith and just beginning to learn about their faith community's beliefs and practices. What are the spiritual requirements for an FCN? The most important requirement is to have a strong faith commitment and be actively involved in your faith community. It is helpful, but not necessary, to have served in faith community leadership roles. Because caring for the spirit is the focus of the faith community and faith community nursing, learning spiritual care skills is very important. Most FCNs will also be involved in the faith community's pastoral care activities, often caring for people in crisis situations, where spiritual care is essential to health and healing.

BASIC PASTORAL CARE FUNCTIONS

There are five basic pastoral care functions that the FCN should keep in mind while working with people:

- Healing: restoring to wholeness
- Sustaining: helping people to endure or transcend their circumstance
- Guiding: assisting with choices
- Reconciling: re-establishing broken relationships
- Nurturing growth

(Reprinted by permission from Clebsch and Jaekle 1964)

PASTORAL CARE

Pastoral care is the ministry of care and counseling provided by spiritual leaders and others to members of their faith community group (church, congregation, etc.). Pastoral care is spiritual accompaniment for people in need, pain, or transition, which includes words and actions that communicate love and concern (Friedman 2001). Through pastoral care, faith community members support one another, especially in times of crisis and struggle.

One aspect of pastoral care is visiting members of the faith community who are lonely, grieving, homebound by age or illness, or receiving care in a hospital or long-term care facility. Judy Glancy, FCN for a large Catholic parish, is an integral part of the faith community's pastoral care. She visits people in their homes and in four hospitals weekly with the help of the priest and deacon. She says this about her role:

> I direct pastoral care in the parish with the assistance of about 15 other parishioners. We visit and take communion and often food to the homebound and those in nursing homes. These visits are most often weekly. I visited an elderly couple weekly for four years, bringing the Eucharist and food from the church freezer made by parishioners. We became good friends. As time went on, Howard became progressively weaker. His diabetes was more out of control and his legs were unable to bear his weight to walk. Orieda and her daughter, Judith, eventually moved a hospital bed into the living room and we assisted them until Howard's death. I then went to their home the day after Howard died and assisted them with planning Howard's funeral, choosing appropriate hymns and readings. I continue to call and visit Orieda while she grieves.

Most FCNs will be involved in visitation and can play an important role, not only in giving spiritual care, but also through ongoing health assessment.

Initially, it may seem somewhat awkward to combine your nursing skills with spiritual care. I clearly remember my first pastoral care visit during my faith community nursing education program. Each FCN was assigned to visit patients in various hospital units. Acting on the chaplain's suggestion, I did not read Mr. Brown's medical chart before my visit. Seated at J.B.'s bedside, I look carefully at him to detect any signs of discomfort. He seems relaxed and comfortable. I think, "He is more comfortable than I am." I scan the room for medical equipment and see none. I wonder what brought him to the hospital. But not having information about his medical condition makes me uneasy. I ask myself, "How can I function as a nurse without this information?" Then I realize I'm not there to perform the usual nursing tasks! I tell Mr. Brown I am from Pastoral Care and ask how he is getting along and if I can do anything for him. I listen as he happily tells me he will be going home soon and then asks me to read from some of his devotional literature. I do that and then, gathering my courage, ask him if he'd like me to pray and what he would like me to pray about. After a short prayer, I say goodbye.

Later that day our class meets to discuss our initial visits. We begin to realize that our ministry role as FCNs is not so much to "do for" people as much as it is to "be with" them. This is part of our discomfort with our new role, feeling like we aren't *doing* anything. Our teacher, Chaplain David Carlson, tells us our primary role in visitation is to listen to a person's story, keeping in mind the unspoken question, "How is it with your soul today?" Initially, this question makes little sense to me. I realize that I have a lot to learn about spiritual care. This may be a new area of learning for you as well. Let's look at some of the resources available to help you gain confidence and skills in this critical component of faith community nursing.

DEVELOPING SPIRITUAL CARE SKILLS

Where do you start in learning spiritual care? You can begin by learning the basics about the theology and practices of the faith community in which you're working. Ask your spiritual leader for guidance, direction, and resources. The spiritual care you give will be unique to your faith community. For example, in Christian faith communities, the FCN may be allowed to perform various spiritual rituals, such as communion or anointing someone with oil for healing. Because you will be representing your faith community in all you do, people will have certain spiritual expectations of you and attach spiritual meaning to your visit. Therefore, learn what type of spiritual care you will be expected and/or allowed to give and find ways to gain the skills and knowledge you need for this important ministry role.

Spiritual care should be a part of every FCN education program. It is an important component of the Parish Nurse Core Curriculum developed by the International Parish Nurse Resource Center (IPNRC). This curriculum is available for use in academic institutions that meet certain criteria. If you do not have access to a program using this curriculum, the IPNRC and the Health Ministries Association have many books and other resources for sale to help you learn spiritual care.

Lay ministry training such as Stephen Ministry may already be available within your faith community. Stephen Ministry is a Christian course led by lay persons that prepares faith community members to care for persons who are in crisis situations. Often faith communities send their FCN for the leadership training needed to serve as a course leader.

Another way to develop spiritual care skills is to enroll in a Clinical Pastoral Education (CPE) program at a nearby healthcare facility. CPE is a standardized program open to seminary students, pastors, and lay persons of all faiths and cultures. Some faith community nursing programs include one unit (400 hours) of CPE. One unit of CPE can also be taken in a 10-week summer program, and CPE programs have been extended over a full year to accommodate working nurses.

Other resources include seminary courses and various types of spiritual formation programs. There are now faith community nursing courses that are part of graduate nursing and seminary education. FCN courses are often available as week-long continuing education offerings. Check the Internet, the IPNRC, and HMA for resources closest to you. Some FCNs pursue a course of study within their larger faith organizations to prepare them for a specialized spiritual role in their faith community, such as a ministry associate or deacon.

In addition to formal preparation in spiritual care, you will want to continue to develop and nurture your own spirit daily. Caring for the spirit in others becomes easier as you care for your own. Taking time to pray or meditate not only fosters your spiritual development and guides you in your work, but it becomes a necessity for your own overall well-being. As a nurse you've experienced how emotionally draining caring for hurting people can be. It is the same in a ministry setting and sometimes more so, because without a time clock to punch, it is harder to set boundaries on your care. Also, in the healthcare setting you had many tools to use. In the ministry setting, the primary tool is yourself.

MINISTRY OF PRESENCE

In your spiritual role you will facilitate healing and growth in people primarily through a ministry of presence, one that involves listening more than speaking (Avery 1986). You'll use the basic communication and counseling skills you learned as a nursing student. Most nurses do not have, and will not need, formal counseling skills to do parish nursing. You might want to review your nursing texts or learn more by reading some pastoral care and counseling texts (see resource list at end of chapter). Your nursing skills and knowledge of relating to hurting people are a great asset in faith community nursing. Because of these, you may be asked to help teach basic counseling and visitation skills to lay visitors.

Most of your informal counseling will involve helping people cope with short-term crises and grief. Rev. Granger Westberg's chaplaincy experience led him to believe that most pastoral care is grief-related in some way. Thus, knowledge of the grief process and ways to help people move through their grief is essential for FCNs.

GRIEF PROCESS

These are the basic tasks of grieving:

- Coming to terms with the reality of loss/death
- Expressing the emotions of loss/death: sadness, anger, relief, guilt, fear
- Using support systems
- Forming a new relationship with the deceased
- Accepting loss
- Making a new beginning: finding new purpose and meaning in life

WAYS TO HELP PEOPLE MOVE THROUGH GRIEF

- Provide a caring presence
- Organize practical help
- Pray with a person
- Encourage spiritual faith
- Listen nonjudgmentally
- Provide information about the grief process and ways to move through it healthfully
- Mobilize support system
- Refer to a professional counselor if needed

To help people in these ways, nurses bring two of the most important qualities with them to faith community nursing: caring and comforting. Caring is providing nursing actions with empathy, and comforting is an action that assists a person to feel better in any dimension. Nurses also have special skills in developing relationships which are essential in giving spiritual care. Nurses know how to establish trusting relationships and are empathetic and good listeners. In listening, you pay attention to a person's story, seeking to hear the meaning they attach to a concern or struggle, how they are coping, and what additional resources you can help them use or access. You will help people identify and use their own personal strengths and resources, including their faith. In my work, I've come to trust that most people know what they need to do to help themselves. They just need others to confirm this in them and support them as they act on their own inner wisdom. In helping people you will, of course, draw on relevant psychodynamic, therapeutic, and theological concepts, and you'll refer people to professional counseling and/or spiritual leaders when psychological or theological issues are beyond your expertise.

Michelle Pearce, a faith community nurse, puts it this way: "I have found that it is my honest and sincere desire to assist people and serve and also the power of Presence that is the most valuable asset that I bring to the church and the people."

INDEPENDENT PRACTITIONER AND MINISTRY TEAM MEMBER

Practicing independently of a healthcare organization may be new to some FCNs who are used to working with other healthcare professionals. In the faith community you will most likely be the only FCN. You may have some nurses, physicians, or other healthcare professionals in the faith community to consult. Depending on the size of the larger community, there may be an abundance of health professionals and agencies or very few. You may be a part of a hospital-sponsored FCN program and have a supervisor and other parish nurses you meet with regularly, or you may have started parish nursing in your faith community on your own. Whatever your situation, remember, you have resources available to you. Other professionals and FCNs are only a phone call or e-mail away.

Faith community nursing is a shared ministry. In thinking of ways to help people, you will always be thinking of how others in the faith community can be involved in meeting someone's need. For example, one of the FCNs in our program connected a lonely elderly man she was visiting with a young woman and her child who then helped him plant his garden. One of your goals will be to help the faith community members minister to one another. You will often be able to connect those wanting to use their gifts in ministry with ministry needs you've identified during home visits. Remember that you do not work alone! Don't forget to pray for divine guidance and direction in your work. Something a spiritual leader reminded me of that was very reassuring and comforting to me in my work as an FCN is that God is already at work in the world and present with people before I arrive.

SPIRITUAL ASSESSMENT

Spiritual assessment is an important part of spiritual care. While much of spiritual assessment will be a gathering of observational data as you work with individuals and groups in the faith community, specific spiritual assessment tools and questionnaires will provide a context for addressing specific spiritual concerns and needs.

Although you may never do a formal spiritual assessment when someone comes to you with a health concern, you'll want to be aware of the ways this concern impacts their spiritual health or whether a spiritual problem might be the basis for the health problem. A physical problem can't help but affect a person's spirit, and a presenting spiritual concern, such as "I just can't pray any more" may mask a psychological concern such as anger or depression. Opportunities for spiritual growth are often missed because people are not encouraged to explore the spiritual roots of their problems (Clinebell 1984).

IMPORTANT ASPECTS OF PHYSICAL AND SPIRITUAL INTERACTIONS

Because body, mind, and spirit are constantly interacting, FCNs must consider all aspects of care. When working with people, keep these questions in mind:

- How does this physical or psychological problem affect this person's spirit?
- How does this spiritual crisis affect this person's body or mind?
- Are any spiritual concerns related to this illness?
- Are spiritual concerns the possible origin of this physical or mental illness?

You'll find helpful information on spiritual assessment in *Nursing the Spirit* (Wilt and Smucker 2001), a practical text for nurses on ways to give spiritual care. A spiritual assessment form that I created for FCNs to use can be found in Appendix A. As people talk about their faith, some will use very concrete terms and stories while others will use more abstract generalizations. Fowler's *Stages of Faith* (Fowler 1981) is useful in identifying how people conceptualize their faith, helping you to know the best ways to talk to them about their faith and use spiritual interventions that will be meaningful to them. Faith, in this developmental model, is the dynamic system of images, values, and commitments that guides one's life. Each progressive stage describes a fundamental set of meanings and values. Although the contents of each stage vary by individuals, the stages progress in the same way from the intuitive, imitative faith of childhood through conventional and then more independent faith to the universalizing, self-transcending faith of full maturity.

USE OF PRAYER AND SCRIPTURE

The spiritual intervention most people will expect from the FCN during a visit is prayer. Even if you have a deeply meaningful personal prayer life, praying out loud is often frightening. It doesn't need to be! If you keep the focus on the person you're visiting and their concerns, prayer will come more easily. Make your prayer personal by praying for people and families by name. You can ask a person if they would like to say a prayer. If they prefer that you pray, ask them what they would like you to pray about. Your prayer does not need to be elaborate. Simply giving their concerns to a transcendent power and asking for that power's healing love, care, and guidance is meaningful to people. Don't be surprised if the person you are praying with cries. Personal prayer touches people deeply, and tears indicate that level of feeling.

In all your work, but especially in using prayer and other faith resources, pray for guidance in choosing what is most appropriate for each person and their situation. Barbara Marlin, FCN in a Lutheran church, gives this example of prayer and praying in her work:

> I met Elizabeth shortly after I started work at the church. She always had a smile, yet at times I sensed a hint of sadness in her eyes. She once shared briefly about losing her husband less than a year before to cancer. I wasn't sure what to do to let her know I was available to her. Of strong German descent, she was very independent. When I suggested a bereavement support group, she told me she was already receiving help from Hospice.
>
> One day a friend of Elizabeth's phoned to let me know Elizabeth was very lonely. Could I call her? I did, and a visit was arranged for that afternoon. I took my Bible and a small vase of pink roses with me. As I drove to the house, I prayed, "Lord, what scripture would you want me to share with her?" The words from Isaiah came to mind: "Fear not, for I have redeemed you...I will be with you...."
>
> As we talked, Elizabeth told me about her growing-up years in Germany, her husband, her child, and grandchildren. Near the close of our visit, I reached for my Bible and said "Elizabeth, on my way here, I was praying for you and what to share. I felt like the Lord laid this scripture on my heart. It's from Isaiah...." Before I could even find the passage, she whispered, "Oh!

My favorite passage is from Isaiah from when I was confirmed as a child in Germany!" I am sure you can imagine the wave of emotion that flooded over her as I began to read the very passage she remembered so well and had clung to all these years. Tears washed her face as I read, then I reached for her delicate hand and shared a prayer of encouragement.

Keep in mind the pastoral counseling guidelines shown below (which I've adapted for parish nurses from Clinebell's classic 1984 text, *Basic Types of Pastoral Care and Counseling*) as you use prayer and other faith resources in your work.

BASIC GUIDELINES FOR USING PRAYER AND FAITH RESOURCES

- Get to know a person's religious background, feelings, and attitudes.
- Before using prayer or other faith resources, ask the person if this would be helpful.
- After using a faith resource, allow people to reflect on what it means to them. This may help them discuss spiritual concerns.
- Faith resources may trigger negative feelings in some people based on past hurtful experiences associated with religion or a faith community.
- Appropriate use of resources should strengthen a person's independence and sense of responsibility, rather than create dependence.
- Include the person's feelings (anger, bitterness, despair) in prayer and choice of resources. This affirms that God accepts human feelings, increases ownership of feelings, and provides an opportunity to release feelings.
- Faith resources are meant to deepen spiritual relationships. Do not use them as a way to avoid relating to the person.
- Be sincere, not mechanical.
- Sometimes no religious words or resources are necessary.
- Inviting people to pray may be more helpful than praying for them.

(Reprinted by permission from Clinebell 1984, pp. 122–23)

Reflecting on my first year of faith community nursing, I realized I was getting frustrated during some of my pastoral visits. Some people seemed to ruminate on past injustices, hurts, or grief, never able to move forward to a point of meaning and gratitude. I knew it was possible for God to transform their pain and for them to experience healing; I just did not know how to help people achieve this. Continuing to just empathically listen to their problems might be digging their emotional rut deeper rather than empowering them to move out of it. If you experience this, one of the things you can do to help people move on is to ask them what is preventing them from putting the pain behind them. In most instances, it is probably a feeling of God's injustice or unfairness. You can reassure them of God's love and presence in their life, but such theological concerns may need to be referred to a professional spiritual leader. If you need help in this area of ministry, I encourage you to talk to an experienced spiritual leader or counselor to learn ways to assist people toward growth and healing. Also, taking time to reflect on your ministry, by yourself or formally with an FCN support group, will enable you to provide more effective spiritual care.

Many FCN groups have used Peter Buttitta's Spiritual Reflection steps (Buttitta 1992) to identify personal and work concerns and gain helpful insights to improve their practice. These steps involve describing the basic facts and feelings related to the concern and then through the use of metaphor and spiritual images gaining insight and clarity which lead to a course of action. For more on this theological reflection method, see Chapter 7.

You may also find spiritual direction helpful in your work. Many faith traditions and cultures have spiritual directors or guides who assist persons to identify where God or their spiritual source is at work in their life and help them interpret what this means for their daily life and work. This guidance may be especially beneficial at the beginning of your ministry or when you experience difficulties.

SUMMARY

Faith community nursing is still a new nursing specialty and many people have never heard of it. One of the most important things you will need to do when starting your practice is to educate the faith community and spiritual leaders about nursing itself, and then about your FCN role. You will get to be creative in the many ways you communicate this information.

For some FCNs, giving spiritual care is a new skill. It is reassuring that nurses already have many of the necessary skills and qualities for ministry. There will be much to learn as an FCN. Not only will you need to be up to date on healthcare knowledge, but you will be learning more about your faith and spiritual care skills. While the FCN is an independent practitioner, remember that you do not work alone. You have many community resources to draw from and you are a member of the ministry team. In thinking of ways to help people, you will always be thinking of how others can be involved in meeting a person's need. Maybe you can connect a person with the pastor, a community agency, or someone in the faith community. Keep the pastoral staff aware of what you're doing, and let them help you develop your role and learn the ways of working in a faith community.

In the next chapter, we'll consider ways to assure good working relationships as you begin your faith community nursing practice.

REFERENCES AND RESOURCES

All online references and resources were current September 30, 2008.

REFERENCES

American Nurses Association and Health Ministries Association. 2005. *Faith community nursing: Scope and standards of practice.* Silver Spring, MD: Nursesbooks.org.

Avery, W. 1986. Toward an understanding of ministry of presence. *The Journal of Pastoral Care* 11 (4):342–53.

Buttitta, P. 1992. *The still, small voice that beckons: A theological reflection method for health ministry.* Chicago: Reflection Resources.

Clebsch, W., and C. Jaekle. 1964. *Pastoral care in historical perspective.* Englewood Cliffs, NJ: Prentice-Hall.

Clinebell, H. 1984. *Basic types of pastoral care and counseling.* Nashville: Abingdon.

Fowler, J. 1981. *Stages of faith.* San Francisco: Harper & Row.

Friedman, D., ed. 2001. *Jewish pastoral care,* 2nd ed. Woodstock, VT: Jewish Lights.

Sawatzky, R., and B. Pesut. 2005. Attributes of spiritual care in nursing practice. *Journal of Holistic Nursing* 23 (1):19–33.

Speck, B. 2003. Undergraduate community health in the first semester: Opportunities and challenges. *Journal of Nursing Education* 42 (7):329–32.

Wilt, D., and C. Smucker. 2001. *Nursing the spirit.* Washington, DC: American Nurses Association.

SUGGESTED RESOURCES

Bradshaw, A. 1994. *Lighting the lamp: The spiritual dimensions of nursing care.* Oxford: Scutari.

Burkhardt, M., and M. Naggai-Jacobsen. 2002. *Spirituality: Living our connectedness.* Albany, NY: Delmar.

Carson, V., and H. Koenig. 2002. *Parish nursing: Stories of service and care.* Philadelphia: Templeton Foundation.

Clark, M., and J. Olson. 2000. *Nursing within a faith community.* Thousand Oaks, CA: Sage.

Clinebell, H. 1984. *Basic types of pastoral care and counseling: Resources for the ministry of healing and growth.* Nashville: Abingdon.

Curtin, L. 1996. This I believe... about the care of human beings. *Nursing Management* 27 (2):5–6.

Dossey, B. 2000. *Holistic nursing: A handbook for practice,* 3rd ed. Gaithersburg, MD: Aspen.

Dossey, L. 1996. *Prayer is good medicine.* San Francisco: Harper.

Hall, B. 1997. Spirituality in terminal illness. *Journal of Holistic Nursing* 15 (1):82–96.

Health Ministries Association. 2002. *A guide to developing a health ministry.* Roswell, GA: Health Ministries Association.

Howe, R. 1963. *The miracle of dialogue.* New York: Seabury.

Lemmer, C. 2002. Teaching the spiritual dimension of nursing care: A survey of U.S. baccalaureate nursing programs. *Journal of Nursing Education* 41 (11):482–90.

McKivergen, M. 1994. The healing process of presence. *Journal of Holistic Nursing* 12(1):65–81.

Nelson, B. 1992. *Igniting the flame: Clinical pastoral education for nurses.* Bristol, PA: Wyndham Hall.

Oates, W. 1971. *The Bible and pastoral care.* Grand Rapids, MI: Baker Book House.

O'Brien, M. 2003. *Parish nursing: Healthcare ministry within the church.* Boston: Jones & Bartlett.

_____. 2000. *Spirituality in nursing: Standing on holy ground.* Mahwah, NJ: Paulist Press.

Shelly, J., ed. 2002. *Nursing in the church.* Madison, WI: InterVarsity Christian Fellowship.

Smucker, C. 1998. Parish nurse programs: Should they include clinical pastoral education? *Perspectives in Parish Nurse Practice (fall issue):*3–5.

Solari-Twadell, P., and M. McDermott, eds. 2005. *Parish nursing: Development, education, and administration.* Philadelphia: Elsevier Mosby.

_____. 1999. *Parish nursing: Promoting whole person health within faith communities.* Thousand Oaks, CA: Sage.

Speck, P. 1988. *Being there: Pastoral care in time of illness.* London: SPCK.

Stanhope, M., and J. Lancaster. 2006. *Foundations of nursing in the community,* 2nd ed. St. Louis: Mosby Elsevier.

Stone, H. 1988. *The word of God and pastoral care.* Nashville: Abingdon.

Taylor, E. 2002. *Spiritual care: Nursing theory, research, and practice.* Upper Saddle River, NJ: Prentice Hall.

Tuck, I., D. Wallace, and L. Pullen. 2001. Spirituality and spiritual care provided by parish nurses. *Western Journal of Nursing Research* 23 (5):441–53.

Wallace, D., I. Tuck, C. Boland, and J. Witucki. 2002. Client perceptions of parish nursing. *Public Health Nursing* 19 (2):128–35.

Westberg, G., and J. McNamara. 1987. *The parish nurse: How to start a parish nurse program in your church.* Park Ridge, IL: Parish Nurse Resource Center.

Whisnant, S. 1999. The parish nurse: Tending to the spiritual side of health. *Holistic Nursing Practice* 14 (1):84–86.

Widerquist, J. and R. Davidhizar. 1994. The ministry of nursing. *Journal of Advanced Nursing* 19 (4):647–52.

ORGANIZATIONAL RESOURCES

American Nurses Association: **www.nursingworld.org**

Association for Clinical Pastoral Education, Inc. (ACPE): **www.acpe.edu**
The ACPE is a multicultural, multi-faith organization devoted to providing education and improving quality of ministry and pastoral care offered by spiritual caregivers of all faiths through the clinical educational methods of Clinical Pastoral Education.

Health Ministries Association: Catalogue of Denominations Resources: **www.hmassoc.org**

International Parish Nurse Resource Center: **www.parishnurses.org**

Intervarsity Christian Fellowship/USA: Books for Parish Nurse Reference: **www.intervarsity.org**

Journal of Pastoral Care: **www.jpcp.org**

Stephen Ministries: **www.stephenministries.org**

CHAPTER 3

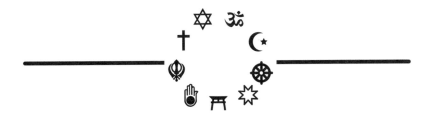

WORKING IN THE FAITH COMMUNITY: THE BASICS

IT'S 9:30 A.M. TUESDAY MORNING and you're attending your first staff meeting. The other staff members there are the two spiritual leaders, organist, and staff associate. The meeting begins with one spiritual leader giving a brief devotion followed by prayer. You think to yourself, "This is a wonderful way to start the work week." Then the meeting begins with a critique of the Sunday worship service: the announcements took too long, the service ran longer than an hour, and the congregation still wasn't singing along with the choir during communion. When the staff asks your opinion, you hesitate to add anything because you are not accustomed to what seems to you as criticizing worship.

EXPECTATIONS

As a new FCN, you're excited about starting to practice where your faith is expected to be a critical component of your work. In fact, you feel that you have been spiritually called to this ministry. You are an active member of a faith community and may serve in a leadership role there. Although some of your experiences as part of a faith community may be negative, probably most of them, like mine, are largely positive. Overall you find the faith community a place of love and support—one that nourishes you and your faith. You probably admire and respect your spiritual leader as a model of faith. From all of these experiences, you bring certain expectations to working in a faith community. Take a moment to think about what they are. Perhaps it will be helpful to write them down so you can reflect on them as you read this chapter. Ask yourself: Are my expectations realistic? How will I deal with unmet expectations?

Your first few weeks in the church will be busy and exciting ones. You will set up your office space, making sure it is easily accessible and private enough to ensure confidentiality. You'll start to get acquainted with the faith community, working hard to remember names and faces. You'll be officially welcomed and start meeting with the program staff and your health committee. There will be an air of excitement in the faith community over the arrival of the new FCN. It will be a thrilling time. As in any new job or relationship, this honeymoon stage will be enjoyable. This period may be heightened in faith community nursing since it is such a new nursing specialty. It brings with it the promise of a more fulfilling practice for the nurse and a new level of well-being for the church. There are many expectations for everyone.

You may first be aware of your own expectations when you see or hear something that doesn't quite fit with what you expected for the faith community. It may be similar to my experience of being asked to critique the worship service. Or it could be a warning to "watch out" for certain people in the faith community or hearing gossip circulating about a staff person's behavior. Somehow you thought the faith community might be protected from the usual workplace politics and problems because it is full of people dedicated to living out their faith.

If you are working in your own faith community, you may be even more shocked and disillusioned when you discover things you weren't aware of as a faith community member. Even if you are not working in your own faith community, you may be surprised that expectations you had of faith communities and spiritual leaders in general are not being met. One reason for these feelings may be because you measure the faith community you're working in by the standards of your own faith community. For example, when I went to a fiftieth wedding anniversary celebration for a couple from the Lutheran church where I was an FCN, I was quite surprised to see the pastor drinking beer! While I learned this was acceptable behavior for Lutheran pastors, I had never seen my Methodist or Presbyterian pastors drinking alcohol publicly. It called into question my previous beliefs about how I expected pastors to behave socially. Later, as coordinator for a Faith Community Nursing Program, new FCNs often reported similar surprises, some of which hurt them deeply. For example, one FCN had only worked a short while before her pastor, whom she loved and respected, left the church over an affair with his secretary.

It is important to consider your expectations and evaluate if they are realistic. Discuss mutual expectations with your supervising spiritual leader early in your ministry. If you have faith community nursing colleagues you regularly meet with, talk with them about their experiences of coming to terms with the realities of working in a church and how they handle the disappointments successfully. It is natural to hold the faith community and its spiritual leadership to higher standards. But it is also important to realize that working in a faith community does not change the fact that we are all human and struggle with the same temptations. We sometimes slip and fall and need forgiveness and reconciliation just like everyone else.

POLITICS

Like a family, the faith community is made up of many different types of people working together to further the faith community's mission. They willingly give their time, energy, and talents for a common goal. To help you understand the dynamics of faith communities, I encourage you to read about family systems. Much of the information, such as family history, secrets, and traditions, will apply and help you understand the family type of dynamics within faith community relationships (Friedman 1985).

You will not be in the faith community long before you'll learn who the lay leaders are. Members will even encourage you to make friends with certain people or avoid others known as "troublemakers." It is true that if the lay leaders in the faith community support you, your work will go easier. But do make your own evaluations rather than prejudging anyone. It will be easier to be objective if you are not a member of the faith community you're working in and do not have any prior allegiances. If this is the case, it will take longer to get to know people and their role in the faith community, but it will put every member on the same basis with you. If you are a member of the faith community, some people may hesitate to confide in you because of who you are friends with. You will have to show them that your friendships will not influence your behavior. In either case, treat everyone the same and maintain strict confidentiality. If people know they can trust you, you have the foundation for good relationships.

Expect that some people in the faith community will try to get their way through political maneuvering or significant financial contributions. Sometimes people who have let it be known that the faith community will receive a large gift after their death unfairly carry more weight in the faith community's decision-making or affect the spiritual leader's behavior and relationships. Also, some people who are tradition-bound oppose change by trying to influence others to their way of thinking. The faith community is not immune to politics. People who work in the faith community can be self-serving and use their influence as leaders to get their way. While you cannot always change these types of behavior in others, you can monitor your own behavior and intentions to ensure that you always act with integrity to keep the faith community's vision and mission on track.

BECOMING PART OF THE TEAM

Not only will you be in a new role by working in a faith community, but having a nurse on the staff may also be a new experience for the ministry team. You'll be learning about their roles, and they'll be learning about yours. But before they can understand what an FCN does, they will often need to know what nurses in general do. You can't assume the staff understands the nursing profession. They are often surprised at the skill set nurses bring to a ministry role, particularly a nurse's ability to relate to people and garner information from them. Although this is an ability most nurses take for granted, it impresses other people.

As you begin to work with the staff, discuss how the FCN will function with the other team members, what tasks will be shared, and how best to integrate faith community nursing activities into the overall program. Initially, the staff may have already made plans for you. For example, when I began as an FCN, I discovered I was already on the calendar to teach a series of health classes on a certain evening. But when the staff held its next planning session, I was a part of it and could then coordinate my activities with theirs. It will take time for the staff to get acquainted with you and to know what ministry areas you can work in independently and in which areas you may need initially to work with others. One example is pastoral visitation. Visitation is often shared among the spiritual leadership staff and lay people. The spiritual leaders may want to know the extent of your experience in visitation and any spiritual training you have had before they allow you to visit members by yourself.

If you are working in a faith community that is not your own, you may discover some differences in beliefs and practices. As an FCN working in a Lutheran congregation, my religious experience (Presbyterian and Methodist) was rooted in a similar Christian Reformed Tradition. Although the beliefs of these three Christian denominations are basically the same, I learned, for example, that the Lutheran beliefs about baptism and confirmation have a different emphasis. Knowing the faith community's beliefs is important as you support and nurture the faith of those in that community and will enable you to better identify spiritual concerns or conflicts that might impact health.

One thing I did that helped me learn more about the faith community's beliefs and practices was to attend a nine-week new members' class. Also, if possible, worship regularly with the faith community and attend other groups and meetings there to learn more about its faith traditions. If you are not practicing in your own faith community, you will need to discuss with your supervisor how often you're expected to attend worship services. Worshiping with the faith community has many benefits for your work. It increases your sense of belonging, makes you more accessible, and enables others to get to know you. However, it does make it difficult to continue to be an active part of your own faith community. As an FCN, I was expected to attend both morning services and an adult education religious class three Sundays a month. Fortunately, my husband was available and willing to take our three children to church. Occasionally, one of my children or the whole family came to worship with me. Though it may be somewhat of a sacrifice, I encourage you to take part in the main worship day activities because I have seen the difference it makes to a faith community nursing practice. Those FCNs who are able and willing to be involved in this way experience their ministry developing more quickly in breadth and depth than those FCNs who are unable to do this.

- Get to know the staff structure and where you fit in it. Knowing the answers to the following questions early in your ministry will help you more quickly become a part of the team.
- How is the staff organized? Is it a hierarchical, independent, or collaborative structure?
- To whom will you report?
- Who approves the faith community nurse's activities?
- What will your relationship be to various committees and the governing body?
- How does the staff communicate with each other? Is it face-to-face informally or by appointment, e-mail, or written memos?

Learn about how the faith community governs itself. Some faith communities have written rules to follow for governance and operation. For example, Presbyterians have their *Book of Order*. Find out if the faith community you're working in has this type of organizational guide and, if so, obtain a copy and use it. Accountability is an important factor in organizational structure and is addressed in Chapter 5.

For a team to work well together, it helps to know your own and others' personality types. There are various personality tools available to help you learn about preferred styles of interacting, processing information, knowing, and decision-making. The Myers-Briggs Type Indicator (MBTI) (Quenk 1999) and the Keirsey-Bates Temperament Sorter (KTS II) are two such tools. Filling out these inventories and discussing them makes for a good continuing education event for staff. These inventories involve choosing your preferred style from a list of various types of situations. Your resulting score identifies your preferred style. Knowing your predominant style gives you a reference point to understand how you interact with others, ways to use your strengths, and how to use your style to work most effectively with others.

When team members respect each other and learn ways to work well together, they not only contribute to the overall quality of the organization, but add joy and satisfaction to work.

LEARNING HOW THINGS ARE DONE: ORGANIZATIONAL CULTURE

The culture of an organization is all the accepted written and unwritten behavioral rules a group of people follow. To work most effectively with your faith community, you will need to learn about its culture and respect the meaning it has for the group.

I learned the hard way about an unwritten rule of visitation: that a church member was to be visited only by the staff member assigned to visit that week. I was in the hospital for some other reason and decided to stop in and say hello to a hospitalized member. I had visited this man in the nursing home and, knowing he was critically ill, thought I should visit him while I was in the hospital. When I told the pastor about my visit, he was not happy. I had broken one of the unwritten rules. On reflection, I could see how multiple staff visits could be confusing to the family and, of course, it wasn't my job that week. Don't be surprised if something like this happens to you. It's not always possible to know all the rules ahead of time.

Having a new person on staff can bring these unwritten rules to light and perhaps suggest a need for a policy manual and/or policy changes. Many faith communities do not have a policy manual. Especially as the size of the staff increases, having written guidelines helps avoid missteps by new employees. As a new employee yourself, you can give valuable input to developing a manual. Someone new sees and experiences things in different ways than someone already familiar with things.

Until you are familiar with how the faith community operates you may need to ask about how to do many things. It surprised me that I had to ask to use certain faith community items in my work. In addition to serving the faith community, I also worked with a couple of neighborhood community agencies supported by the faith community. At a food bank, I took weekly blood pressure readings for people. Later, to serve more people, I did the same thing at a grocery store across the street. To do this I needed to borrow the church's card table and a couple of folding chairs. I'd worked for the faith community long enough at that point to know that I even needed to ask permission to use these things outside the church. It just takes time to learn what you can and cannot do. When in doubt—ask!

Another example of learning how things are done is when I planned to take blood pressure readings after the church services and enlist the help of other nurses. Based on my own faith community experience, I assumed that more people would attend the later morning worship service and I would need to schedule more nurses for that one. But in discussing my plans with my supervising pastor, I learned that the earlier morning service had the larger attendance. In other words, you can't assume things are the same in each faith community. Which service most people attend is just one part of the organizational culture you'll need to understand.

Even if you are working in your own faith community, there will be ways of doing things you will not know unless you ask the administrative assistants. Your work will go smoother if they become your friends early on. You'll need to know how much, if any, administrative support you'll have and which person will assist you with your work. As more faith community staffs use computers, they tend to do most of their own writing. But you will still need to know things like the newsletter deadline and how much space you have in it. Often these support staff have worked for the faith community many years under several different spiritual leaders. Not only can they tell you how to operate the equipment, such as copiers, but they know the format and deadlines for everything, including the church calendar. They also have a wealth of information about the history, tradition, and culture of the faith community that will be invaluable to your work. The faith community calendar is often found in the administrative office with all faith community events posted on it. When planning programs, consult this calendar frequently. Outside groups may also use the building, so knowing when other groups meet and which rooms they use will avoid scheduling conflicts.

CULTURAL COMPETENCY

Ideally, the FCN's cultural background is matched to that of the faith community. However, that is not always possible, and the people you are working with may have a culture different from your own. Even if your cultures are similar, you may be working with different cultures through working with the faith community's outreach ministries. Two of the FCNs in our program worked with the homeless as a part of the weekly meal served for them at the church. Another FCN, who was Caucasian, served an inner-city African–American faith community. Later she worked with an inner-city youth foundation doing health teaching and assisting juvenile first offenders learn healthier ways of living. In all these situations, the FCNs had to learn about the different cultures of the people plus the culture of poverty, minorities, and the homeless. Understanding cultural characteristics is essential to giving quality care.

To begin to learn about these cultures, collecting information using a cultural assessment tool may be helpful. Doing a cultural assessment is an important part of your initial and ongoing assessment of the faith community. Included in a cultural assessment are the ways people communicate with each other, their preferred amount of personal space, how they celebrate significant life events, and their perceptions of time and environmental control (Lester 1998).

Another essential cultural understanding for a faith community nurse is knowing the meaning people give to health and illness and what types of self-care are practiced. For instance, do people attribute illness to broken relationships or as punishment for sin? Do they use folk medicine of any kind? These are important questions to ask as you do health counseling. Also, knowing what a cultural group's experience has been with the healthcare system may help you understand their attitude toward it and also their use of it. For example, because of the way African–Americans have historically been treated, they often distrust health care. Knowing this, you can provide more education to help this group seek and accept medical treatment when needed. To learn more about cultural differences, talk to faith community members and utilize relevant print and visual media.

The following two examples show that the better you understand the culture, the more effective your ministry will be.

> Jennifer Simpson worked at a Blacksburg, Virginia, mosque while she was a nursing graduate student at Radford University. She had converted to Islam and later married a Muslim from Jordan. She kept office hours twice a week in the mosque to counsel and advise patients. She calls this version of faith community nursing *crescent nursing*. Simpson's care takes into consideration the cultural and language

differences and a lack of communication and awareness about healthcare services that are barriers to Muslims acquiring medical care. She says, "There is a desperate need for culturally sensitive health programs and culturally sensitive healthcare providers." Her goal is to improve the quality of life for Muslims, especially women, by providing language-specific informational programs about preventative care such as breast self-exams, family planning, and annual screening for cervical and breast cancers (Zinkle 2003).

Linda Weinberg, PhD, RN, NP, ET, serves as a Jewish congregational nurse through Jewish Family and Children's Service and her synagogue in the Philadelphia area. Her background as a family nurse practitioner and as a Jewish chaplain guides her work. One cultural example from her work relates to meeting a person's spiritual need:

> When I tried to change the man's wound dressings, he resisted, locking himself in the bedroom. After speaking with his wife, she discovered the man was grieving over the anniversary of his mother's death. The elderly man wanted to say Kaddish, a prayer usually said in synagogue, that demonstrates the highest love to honor and remember a deceased relative. Because the man was too sick to go to synagogue, Linda said Kaddish with him before dressing his wounds.

Linda says there are other ways a Jewish congregational nurse can be uniquely helpful. For example, the nurse can advise a Jewish patient with hypertension to modify kosher foods in the diet that are heavy in salt (Coleman 2002). (Read more about Linda's Model of Jewish Congregational Nursing in Chapter 8.)

The principal cultural characteristics that an FCN needs to assess to provide appropriate and acceptable health care are listed in the adjacent sidebar.

Cultural Considerations

- Preferred title
- Immigration history
- Communication style
- Personal space
- Celebrations
- Life and death rituals
- Activities of daily living
- Food practices
- Symptom management
- Family relationships
- Illness beliefs
- Health practices
- Perceptions of time and control

PREVENTING AND RESOLVING CONFLICT

Whenever people work together, it's possible for some type of conflict to occur because of differences in personality, work style, or education. Most likely one of the earliest conflicts, and most important to resolve, may be between you and your supervisor, who is usually one of the spiritual leaders of the faith community. In this relationship, conflict may arise because of the differences in your preparation for ministry. If the spiritual leader knows you as a member of the faith community, he or she may already be aware of and confident in your spiritual care skills. Otherwise, it may take some time before you will be allowed to do certain things, such as visitation, on your own.

Assess your spiritual care skills. What is your background in ministry? How can you better prepare yourself for the spiritual part of your role? In addition to the resources listed in Chapter 2, take time each day to grow in the knowledge and practice of your faith. Your ministry credibility will grow naturally, too, as your supervisor sees your knowledge and skills at work and the ways faith community nursing supports and complements the faith community's mission and ministry.

However, in faith communities where women do not regularly serve in leadership roles, the female FCN may experience some discrimination. Although serving in her own faith community, one FCN was surprised, and somewhat offended, by having to meet with the support staff rather than the program staff. AN FCN may also be excluded from weekly program staff meetings because of a non-paid or part-time status and can address this issue in an interview. One of the questions a female FCN can ask the interview committee is, "How will a female staff person be accepted by this faith community, including both the congregation and the leadership or pastoral staff?" Knowing such information about a faith community before you take the position of FCN there can help avoid hurt feelings and possible conflict.

Things to Consider Before Accepting a Position in a Faith Community

- Are my beliefs compatible with the faith community's?
- Do I agree with the faith community's mission?
- Is my nursing background a good match for the health needs and ministries of this faith community?
- Will my personality be a good fit with the personalities of the staff?
- Will any of my personal characteristics (race, age, economic status) interfere with my ministry?
- What are the faith community's required qualifications for leadership roles?
- What is the faith community's stance on issues such as abortion?
- Am I willing and able to also work in the community surrounding the church if asked?
- Does my experience match the specific age groups and/or ministries to which I'll be assigned, such as the homeless or inner-city populations?

Another possible conflict between you and your supervisor may occur as you and your accomplishments become well known and valued in the faith community. You may even feel as though you have been put on a pedestal. Initially that feels pretty good, but it's probably a new experience for you and perhaps an unwelcome one. Your popularity may threaten some spiritual leaders who, consequently, may act out their feelings by being overly controlling or critical of your work. If this is the case, talk about it directly with them as soon as possible.

It is essential for you to meet regularly with your supervisor to keep lines of communication open, to share ideas about the best ways to meet the health-related needs of the congregation, and to integrate your work into the overall ministry. Forming a good working relationship with your supervisor is a process that begins with a commitment to trust and respect each other. It involves valuing each other's differences and a willingness to learn from each other.

As you work in these ways to create a collegial and collaborative relationship with your supervisor, the following tool may be helpful. The *Ministry Partnership Continuum* is a model which identifies the elements of relationships (such as gender and education differences) and enables the senior spiritual leader and FCN to move from *stereotyping* to *transition* and finally to *power equity*. Discussing these and other relationship elements (for example, worldviews of wholistic health care and spirituality, nurse and clergy identity) may help senior spiritual leaders and FCNs dialogue about their relationship, how they experience it, and thus develop a relationship of mutual respect and trust (Clark 2000; pp. 300–304; Pierce, Page, and Wagner, 1998).

To have good relationships and prevent conflict with other faith community staff, get to know them and what they do. One way to do this is to obtain copies of their job descriptions if they are available. Always support their activities and plan your work with the total faith community program in mind. Each staff person has his or her area of expertise. The FCN must be aware of the delicate balance between sharing ministry and perceived turf issues. Learn your ministry boundaries. This is where having a clear job description for yourself as an FCN is helpful. A job description serves to clarify your role and communicate it to others. It can also be used as an evaluation tool to measure your performance. If you are a part of a hospital-sponsored program, your job description may be provided for you. If not, write your own in consultation with the spiritual leader and your health committee using *Faith Community Nursing: Scope and Standards of Practice* as a guide.

Although conflict cannot always be avoided, by knowing the potential areas where it might erupt, you can lay the groundwork for conflict prevention and resolution. Communication is probably the most important way to avoid and resolve conflict. Keep things out in the open. When you feel a problem is brewing, deal with it directly and open it up to discussion.

MINISTRY BOUNDARIES

Each staff person has his or her area of responsibility. Get acquainted with each person's area. In a faith community, some ministries may overlap. You will need to know your area so you won't encroach on someone else's territory. Don't overstep your ministry boundaries. Especially remember you are not the senior spiritual leader! For example, your visits to members do not take the place of the spiritual leader's visits. Usually your visitation assignment will be made by the senior spiritual leader. If a member comes up to you and asks you to visit her or one of her friends or family members, obtain the person's permission and then talk with the senior spiritual leader before responding immediately to that need. You may find that the need is already being taken care of by others, or the spiritual leader may want someone else to attend to that need or work with you. As you assess the faith community's needs, again talk to the senior spiritual leader and other staff before going ahead with your plans. Visitation parameters and confidentiality issues need to be clarified for any FCN.

What to Include in a Job Description

- FCN qualifications (e.g., education, experience, licensure)
- Person the FCN reports to
- Job summary

Areas of responsibility according to *Faith Community Nursing: Scope and Standards of Practice* (ANA and HMA 2005)

Guidelines for Working in the Faith Community

- Identify your expectations before beginning work in the faith community.
- Evaluate your expectations periodically. Keep them realistic.
- Follow your job description and maintain ministry boundaries.
- In establishing relationships, maintain confidentiality and build on a foundation of trust.
- When in doubt, ask.
- Communicate. Communicate. Communicate.
- Learn about the faith community: its history, culture, government, structure, and family dynamics.
- Establish a health committee and meet with it regularly.
- Meet regularly with your supervisor and other staff.
- Learn from your experiences.

Federal privacy rules under the 1996 Health Insurance Portability and Accountability Act (HIPAA) apply to faith community nursing. In general, the rules require healthcare providers to limit disclosure of personal health information to the *minimum necessary* for a particular purpose. The law says reasonable steps must be taken to keep patient information private. HIPAA is also discussed in relationship to collaboration and ethics in Chapter 5.

Although you are eager to spread the word about faith community nursing, some groups may be considered off-limits for this presentation. In my case, it was the women's circles, because their primary purpose was Bible study. Because I wanted to get acquainted with as many people as possible, I decided to just attend each circle meeting and then schedule women's programs at other times. Again, it's a part of getting to know the faith community you are in and the ways they do things.

As you make friends in the faith community, people may want you to take sides with them on a faith community issue or complain to you about others on the staff. Listen to them but encourage them to address their concern directly to the person involved. Do not agree with them or pass the information on to others. Nothing will destroy your relationship with the other staff members sooner than undermining someone's ministry in this way. Be very clear in letting people know that you support the staff and that you will not align yourself with one faction or another.

Sometimes faith community conflicts may involve your ministry. The health committee can be very helpful to you when a conflict arises between you and either the staff or the faith community. If you are unable to resolve a disagreement yourself, your health committee may be able to intervene. In one situation I was involved in as the FCN's supervisor, the faith community committee responsible for including the FCN's salary in its budget decided on its own to eliminate the FCN position to get its budget in line with recommendations. The real problem was that the group didn't know all the ways the faith community nursing ministry was helping people in the church. Because the FCN felt uncomfortable dealing with this problem alone, I spoke with the Health Committee chairperson who understood the importance of faith community nursing. He wrote a letter to the committee, convincing them to retain the FCN position but place it more appropriately under the Personnel Committee. By building a solid health committee, one that is up to date on your activities and assists with your program, you will have an invaluable support system and ally in times of conflict. Also, if you are part of a hospital-sponsored program, always inform your program supervisor of any emerging problem. Part of your supervisor's job is to help you in this type of situation.

CHANGE IN FAITH COMMUNITY LEADERSHIP

Some faith communities change leadership infrequently, while others change every few years. When a change occurs, a new senior spiritual leader may be in place immediately or not for several years. During this time an interim senior spiritual leader may be assigned. These transition periods can sometimes be very difficult times for the faith community and staff. You may suddenly not have a supervisor, the faith community may be in turmoil, and everyone may take sides. The interim senior leader may know nothing about faith community nursing and not have the time to learn about it because just holding the faith community together is the main concern. During these times, the FCN often serves as the glue that holds the community together. When a new senior leader arrives, your help will be invaluable. You can provide information not only about your own work but also about the needs of the community. With new leadership comes uncertainty about whether your position will continue. Again, your health committee can support your position by informing the new senior leader about how your ministry has affected the community's health and wholeness and how it contributes to the overall ministry and mission.

LIABILITY AND INSURANCE

Whether you are working as a paid or unpaid FCN, you must adhere to all state and local nursing regulations and maintain an active nursing license. I also recommend that you carry liability insurance. Even though faith community nurses do not usually give medications or perform medical procedures, there are aspects of their care—such as giving health advice and maintaining confidentiality—that are vulnerable to litigation.

Liability issues are some of the biggest concerns for faith communities considering faith community nursing. It is a good idea for the faith community to inform its insurance carrier that it has an FCN on staff and, if necessary, add a rider to the policy to cover the FCN. Some faith community insurance policies as well as nursing liability policies now include coverage for FCNs. If they do not yet have this category, select the category, such as educator, that best describes your primary FCN role.

If you are covered by a hospital's liability policy as a hospital employee (if your FCN salary and benefits are paid directly by the hospital) seek legal advice to learn whether carrying your own liability policy is in your best interest.

You may discover other legal concerns or issues as you practice. One that affected our FCNs was when the hospital lab did health screening tests at faith community sites. New state regulations required a physician to interpret the test results before an FCN could report them to the people tested. The FCNs often found a physician in the faith community or on their health committee willing to help in this way.

DOCUMENTATION ·

Since record-keeping is a required legal accounting of nursing care, what should the FCN be documenting? That will depend on the types of things you do as an FCN. For FCNs who focus on teaching health classes and conducting blood pressure screenings, keeping blood pressure records will be the major record-keeping required. Blood pressure records should include: a list of people served, the screening dates, the blood pressure numbers, and the dates you made follow-up calls to individuals with high blood pressure. If your practice includes visitation, you'll want to record health assessment data, your interventions, and other significant information as part of the nursing process.

To minimize the amount of time you spend documenting, design a system that meets the expected standards while being most efficient for you. You can record this information on an index card or in a computer file. Some FCNs use laptop computers on home visits and input data after each visit. Choose a healthcare documentation format that meets your needs (see Chapter 4 for suggested systems). Computer software for faith community nursing has been under development and may now be available. If your practice is part of a healthcare system, you may be required to use its clinical record forms, which are legally the system's property. That means that if you leave the faith community, the records will be kept by the healthcare system, not the faith community.

To ensure confidentiality, keep your paper files in a locked file cabinet and ensure that your computer files can be accessed only by you. You can do your monthly reports on your computer. If your supervisor requires a copy, they can be easily sent as an e-mail attachment. Careful documentation also helps researchers study your practice. Using computers for documentation is helpful because they are password protected and information is backed up on a disk which can be locked up to maintain confidentiality.

End-of-year reports, such as the faith community's annual report, are another way of communicating what you do, as well as an accountability measure. Be sure you are included in this and other faith community reporting.

REIMBURSEMENT

Many FCNs give their time voluntarily, on an unpaid basis as a ministry to their faith community. This type of service has a long and valuable history. However, if you expect your ministry to grow and become a vital part of your faith community's ministry, you should from the beginning put it on a professional basis by being paid, if only for the resources you use. Just because your faith community is small, don't think it can't provide you with some financial reimbursement, perhaps just mileage reimbursement for your home visits. From my experience, if the faith community values your professional service, it will find the money for the ministry. Although your ministry may be funded initially by one faith community member's gift or an outside grant, your ministry will be more valued and visible if it is a line-item in the faith community's operational budget. When people know they are contributing financially to the ministry, they will naturally be more aware of and interested in it. In other words, they will have a sense of ownership in it. And as they see your documented results and experience your care, they will begin to see the value of your health ministry work.

For a faith community to invest in a new ministry such as faith community nursing requires a step of faith. Rarely does a faith community understand initially the many ways this ministry will enhance its overall ministry until an FCN actually begins work. Be sure to point out the ways faith community nursing contributes to the faith community's mission. This information can make health ministry seem more relevant to the faith community until they experience other aspects of faith community nursing and appreciate its relevance for themselves.

When faith community nursing began in the 1980s, several foundations, such as the Lutheran Wheatridge Foundation, were eager to fund this new venture. However, once faith community nursing spread across the country and became an established nursing specialty, grant funding diminished. Most foundations today want to fund projects primarily in their beginning stages to get them off the ground or to fund new creative ideas, particularly collaborative programs in which a variety of community agencies work together. The most likely grant funding for faith community nursing now comes from within specific faith group foundations, foundations within your geographic area, or a large foundation, such as the Templeton Foundation, which supports a variety of spiritual projects, most recently research on forgiveness, spiritual care curricula in nursing education, and a book on faith community nursing. Many books are available on grant writing to help you put a proposal together (see Suggested Resources at end of the chapter). Since writing a proposal is a time-consuming project, first contact the foundation or consult a book listing foundations to find out what type of projects they typically fund.

BUDGET

Even before you begin as an FCN in a faith community, you need to have some idea of what the ministry will cost annually. I've always suggested to faith communities that they set aside at least $1,000 for the faith community nurse ministry (in addition to salary and benefits, if provided). This is a good beginning amount to cover the basic resources (see sidebar) needed for various activities. During the year, keep track of what you spend so that you'll have some basis for creating next year's budget. Some faith communities ask you to account for every piece of paper, while others want to know only an overall estimate of major expenses and the cost of future activities. Each faith community will handle its budget process differently. What is most important is that the faith community nursing ministry is a part of the budget. Find out how your church puts its budget together and see that you are included in the process.

Typical Budget Expenses

- Office supplies (printer paper, file folders, etc.)
- Teaching materials (PowerPoint slides, overhead transparencies, handouts)
- Blood pressure equipment
- Refreshments (served at programs)
- Thank-you gifts for volunteers
- Business cards
- Signs (purchased or materials to make your own)
- Reference books
- Health books for faith community library

SUMMARY

Beginning a faith community nursing ministry in a church is exciting and fulfilling. You will have both hopes and fears. Most likely, your hopes will exceed your expectations and many of your fears will never be realized. However, difficulties can arise because faith community nursing is new to many people and because each faith community is made up of human beings! Many experiences, such as political maneuvering, may surprise and even shock the new FCN. By learning where the potential dangers are, establishing a viable health committee, and becoming a trusted member of the ministry team through open communication, many conflicts can be avoided or resolved. Also, by taking a serious look at liability and reimbursement issues, creating a budget, and planning your method of documentation, you will establish your practice on a solid foundation to assure its future success.

REFERENCES AND RESOURCES

All online references and resources were current September 30, 2008.

REFERENCES

American Nurses Association and Health Ministries Association. 2005. *Faith community nursing: Scope and standards of practice.* Silver Spring, MD: Nursesbooks.org.

Clark, M.. 2000. Nurses and faith community leaders growing in partnership. In M. Clark and J. Olson, eds., *Nursing within a faith community,* pp. 297–316. Thousand Oaks, CA: Sage.

Coleman, S. 2002. Finding new ways to serve. *Advance Online Editions for Nurses.* King of Prussia, PA: Merion Publications.

Friedman, E. 1985. *Generation to generation: Family process in church and synagogue.* New York: Guildford.

Lester, N. 1998. Cultural competence: A nursing dialogue. *American Journal of Nursing* 98 (8): 26–34.

Pierce, C., B. Page, and D. Wagner. 1998. *A male/female continuum: Paths to colleagueship.* Laconia, NH: New Dynamics.

Zinkle. 2003. Crescent support helps Muslims–Nursing. *USA Today* (Society for the Advancement of Education/Gale Group), October 2003.

SUGGESTED RESOURCES

Brewer, E., C. Achilles, J. Fuhriman, and C. Hollingsworth. 2001. *Finding funding: Grantwriting from start to finish, including project management and Internet Use,* 4th ed. Newbury Park, CA: Corwin Press.

Chase-Ziolek, M. 2005. *Health, healing, and wholeness: Engaging congregations in ministries of health.* Cleveland, OH: Pilgrim.

Chase-Ziolek, M., and L. Holst. 2000. Parish nursing in diverse traditions. In A. Solari-Twadell and M. McDermott, eds., *Parish nursing: Promoting whole person health within faith communities,* pp. 195–204. Thousand Oaks, CA: Sage.

Clark, M. 2000. Characteristics of faith communities. In M. Clark and J. Olson, *Nursing within a faith community,* pp. 17–27. Thousand Oaks, CA: Sage.

Djupe, A. 1990. Adjustments, myths, and realities of parish nursing. In M. McDermott, A. Djupe, and A. Solari-Twadell, eds., *Parish nursing: The developing practice,* Chapter 9. Park Ridge, IL: International Parish Nurse Resource Center.

Elfrink, V., S. Bakken, A. Coeenen, B. McNeil, and C. Bickford. 2001. Standardized nursing vocabularies: A foundation for quality care. *Seminars in Oncology* 12 (1): 18–23.

Engebretson, J., and J. Headley. 2000. Cultural diversity and care. In B. Dossey, et al., eds., *Holistic nursing: A handbook for practice,* 3rd ed., pp. 283–310. Gaithersburg, MD: Aspen.

Fite, R. 1999. The congregation as a workplace. In A. Solari-Twadell and M. McDermott, eds., *Parish nursing: Promoting whole person health within faith communities,* pp. 123–33. Thousand Oaks, CA: Sage.

Giger, J., and R. Davidhizer. 2004. *Transcultural nursing: Assessment and intervention,* 4th ed. St. Louis: Mosby.

Gitlin, L., and K. Lyons. 2003. *Successful grant writing: Strategies for health and human service,* 2nd ed. New York: Springer.

Hall, M., and S. Howlett. 2003. *Getting funded: The complete guide to writing grant proposals,* 4th ed. Portland, OR: Portland State University.

Health Ministries Association. 2004. *A guide to developing a health ministry.* Roswell, GA: HMA.

Huff, R., and M. Kline, eds. 1998. *Promoting health in multicultural populations: Handbook for practitioners.* Thousand Oaks, CA: Sage.

Kenner, C., and M. Walden. 2001. *Grant writing tips for nurses and other health professionals.* Washington, DC: American Nurses Publishing.

Kim-Godwin, Y., P. Clarke, and L. Barton. 2001. A model for the delivery of culturally competent community care. *Journal of Advanced Nursing* 35 (6): 918–25.

Leininger, M. 1991. *Culture care diversity and universality: A theory of nursing.* New York: National League for Nursing.

——. 2002. Culture care assessments for congruent competency practices. In M. Leininger and M. McFarland, eds., *Transcultural nursing: Concepts, theories, research, and practice*, 3rd ed., pp. 117–43. New York: McGraw-Hill.

Lipson, J., S. Dibble, and P. Minarik, eds. 1996. *Culture and nursing care: A pocket guide.* San Francisco: University of California School of Nursing, UCSF Nursing Press.

Maranto, G. 2002. Overcoming cultural barriers for better care. *New York Times.com,* October 1, 2002.

Marshall, E. 1999. *Building trust at the speed of change: The power of the relationship-based corporation.* New York: AMACOM.

Patterson, D. 2003. *Essential parish nurse: ABCs for congregational health ministry.* Cleveland, OH: Pilgrim.

Purnell, L., and B. Paulanka. 2004. *Guide to culturally competent health care.* Philadelphia: F.A. Davis.

Quenk, N. 1999. *Essentials of Myers-Briggs type indicator assessment.* New York: John Wiley & Sons.

Richardson, R. 1996. *Creating a healthier church: Family systems theory, leadership, and congregational life.* Minneapolis, MN: Fortress.

Shen, Z. 2004. Cultural competence models in nursing: A selected annotated bibliography. *Journal of Transcultural Nursing* 15 (4): 317–22.

Spector, R. 2004. *Cultural diversity in health and illness,* 6th ed. Upper Saddle River, NJ: Pearson Prentice Hall.

Tuck, I., and D. Wallace. 2000. Exploring parish nursing from an ethnographic perspective. *Journal of Transcultural Nursing* 11 (4): 290–99.

Vandecreek, L., ed. 2001. Chaplains, clinical pastoral education supervisors, parish nurses, and community clergy in relationship. *Journal of Health Care Chaplaincy* 11 (2): 1–98.

Wallace, D., I. Tuck, C. Boland, and J. Witucki. 2002. Client perceptions of parish nursing. *Public Health Nursing* 19 (2): 128–35.

Organizational Resources

The Alban Institute: **www.alban.org.** An ecumenical, interfaith organization supporting congregations through consulting services, research, book publishing, and educational seminars.

Journal of Transcultural Nursing: **www.tcns.org** (Transcultural Nursing Society)

The Keirsey-Bates Temperament Sorter (KTS II) is available on the Web at
keirsey.com/cgi-bin/keirsey/newkts.cgi

Myers-Briggs Type Indicator: **www.humanmetrics.com**

Stephen Ministries Program (lay ministry training): **www.stephenministries.org**

CHAPTER 4

INTEGRATING FAITH AND HEALTH USING STANDARDS OF PRACTICE

> When our priest asked me to co-lead a grief support group with our pastoral care coordinator, the coordinator and I reviewed the material that the previous group leaders had used. We decided to use it again because of its sound psychological basis. But as we talked together about the grief process, our faith, and the role of the faith community in health and healing, we asked each other, "Why isn't there a spiritual component to this curriculum?" Realizing this, we added several spiritual elements: memorial candles to create a worship atmosphere, opening and closing prayer, and Bible readings and prayers that related to each weekly theme

INTEGRATING FAITH AND HEALTH through the intentional care of the spirit sets faith community nursing apart from other nursing specialties. Michelle Pearce, FCN, clearly identifies this as her main goal: "My ministry has been one primarily of wholism, helping people to integrate body–mind–spirit, finding ways for people to bring their faith into their daily lives and health practices and dying experiences." Although this integration is challenging to achieve, your efforts will be rewarded as you begin to see people make this connection themselves. While talking with a woman about her health history before she joined the weight management program I started as an FCN, I asked about recent life events. She told me, "My daughter just got divorced." As I listened to what this meant to her, she began to connect this event to her recent feelings of stress and current health concerns. When people don't make these connections themselves, you can help them do so by explaining how psychological, emotional, or spiritual pain affects overall health and may lead to physical problems. As you engage people in this type of wholistic dialogue they will gradually begin to think this way themselves, becoming more aware of how all they do affects health and what they need to do to achieve wholeness.

A rather dramatic example of this occurred when a friend of mine was telling me about the current stress in her life and her recent physical problems. She said, "I know that all these things have a physical effect on me. I'm concerned about some physical manifestations. I get an upset stomach, or I wake up in the morning with a headache. I can think of three particular incidents where something was happening that I just couldn't stand and then that's the way I'd express it. I had lower back pain and I couldn't stand up straight. And then another time I wanted to tell someone something that bothered me and I just couldn't bring myself to do it—and I got laryngitis and couldn't talk. And then there was the time when my husband was pushing me through some project and my neck started hurting—a pain in the neck, you know. A couple of years ago I felt like I needed a break, and, well, I broke my leg." She finished by saying, "I've seen those things happen to myself and I'm concerned. I just feel like all these things are killing me." As soon as those words were out of her mouth, she sat back, amazed at what she had said. Connecting her physical problems to what she identified as "her soul's sickness" was an insight that was a turning point for her and motivated her to make some necessary changes in her life.

Ten years later she called to thank me again for listening to her that day and to tell me how what she had learned about herself was helping her through her present difficulty. Listening is a precious gift you give people and a powerful tool for change. Helping people to thoughtfully reflect on their situation may lead to life-changing insights.

Rev. Granger Westberg talks about those people in the faith community, like my friend above, who are "a little bit sick." These are the ones whose "early cries for help" he believes FCNs can hear and attend to. The cry that he heard most frequently in his work as a hospital chaplain was grief. Most of what happens in life, he says, whether good or bad, includes the experience of loss and thus grief. For example, welcoming a new baby into your home is usually a happy event. However, it is associated with various common losses: sleep, individual freedom, and for a woman, at least temporarily, her figure. Rev. Westberg believes that many illnesses can be prevented if grief and loss are addressed when they first occur.

What other ways can you help people make these faith and health connections? As mentioned in Chapter 2, you will have many opportunities to tell people from the very beginning of your ministry about this central faith community nursing focus. Another way is to make your teaching wholistic whenever possible. When I began as an FCN, the staff had already designated a six-week period for me to teach "something on health." With only a month to prepare, I chose health topics with which I had the most up-to-date knowledge and experience: cancer, depression, and cardiovascular health. Although I opened and closed the sessions with prayer, I did not even think to relate current science to religious beliefs and practice. There were probably several reasons for this. In 1986, little research had examined this relationship, and the faith community nursing role was just beginning to be defined. Not only was I not quite sure about all that I was supposed to be doing—neither was the faith community. The good news is that these things have changed significantly since then.

The number of research studies being done on the health effects of such spiritual variables as prayer, meditation, faith commitment, and forgiveness continues to increase. Almost every day you see results of these studies in the media. Some organizations such as the Templeton Foundation fund only research which studies the faith–health connection. The work of the former National Institute for Healthcare Research (Larson, Swyers, and McCullough 1998) contributed significantly to our understanding of the relationship between faith and health by analyzing research studies on health which contained spiritual variables. The National Center for Complementary and Alternative Medicine (NCCAM) conducts research on many types of complementary and alternative therapies including mind–body interventions such as meditation (www.nccam.nih.gov).

As I realized the importance of integrating faith and health in my faith community nursing role, I looked for religious materials to help me make these connections in my teaching. I found a study on *Ministries of Healing* (Daehling and Soder-Alderfer 1984) that I used as a six-week adult education class; later I led a four-part series based on the Tubesings' book *The Caring Question* (1983), which explores the balance between caring for others and self-care (now published as *Seeking Your Healthy Balance* 1991). For group activities, I found the Tubesings' book, *Structured Exercises in Wellness Promotion* (1986/1994), useful as group icebreakers and discussion starters that supported the wholistic health principles presented in classes.

Today, many such resources are available. Many publishers of religious materials develop teaching materials specifically for faith community health ministries. These materials address the role of the faith community in health and healing as well as the ways the faith community can care for people dealing with specific health issues such as mental illness, AIDS, and disabilities. Check out your own faith community's resources as well as local libraries, bookstores, and the Internet. If you want to use materials from other faiths, be sure the theological perspective is similar to that of the faith community in which you're working. If it differs, talk with the senior spiritual leader and/or religious educator on staff regarding the most appropriate way to use the material.

Even if the material's theological point of view is consistent with the faith community's, be aware that people within the faith community may hold diverse theological views. One FCN discovered this when she used a spiritually based weight management program that another FCN had used successfully in her faith community. Although the program had been approved by the second faith community's staff, some of the class members found the underlying theology disturbing. The FCN took time to discuss the theological differences with the class, and since overall the class found the material helpful, they decided to continue using the materials.

Working to integrate faith and health in all you do as an FCN will be challenging. The field of disease prevention and health promotion itself is still developing. Increasing amounts of information will be available to help you do this in the faith community. By using a variety of resources, you will find creative ways to present this information to people and help them implement it in their lives. For ideas, find other professionals in your community who are working in these same areas.

You can contribute to further developments in this field yourself by assisting with research in the areas of faith and health. This research may eventually validate scientifically personal experiences of receiving comfort and healing through faith. It is an exciting time to be a part of these efforts. Don't underestimate how much you can contribute to the growing understanding of health and healing from your knowledge and experience as an FCN.

FAITH COMMUNITY NURSING FUNCTIONS

You will weave faith and health into your practice through the various functions you perform as an FCN. Rev. Granger Westberg identifies these four functions in his original book on parish nursing (1987):

• Health educator

• Personal health counselor

• Trainer of volunteers

• Organizer of support groups

The first two functions are ones most nurses use every day in practice and the ones we've talked about so far in this book. The third one, training volunteers, is important since faith communities are primarily volunteer organizations. We'll talk about working with volunteers in Chapter 6.

There are now seven functions that are considered essential to faith community nursing practice. These additional functions (and where they are discussed in this book) are:

• Integrator of faith and health (in Chapter 4),

• Referral agent (in Chapter 4)

• Health advocate (in Chapters 4 and 5).

You may discover there are other functions needed in your particular faith community nursing practice.

As an FCN you may be involved with support groups in some way since faith communities often help people deal with life issues through groups such as for grief or addictions. If you are asked to lead a group or train others to lead one, you'll need skills in small group leadership in addition to those skills you already have in teaching and counseling.

In response to the results of my initial congregational survey of health needs and interests, I started two support groups: a weight management group for women and a caregiver's group for those caring for an elderly relative. The weight management group did not continue beyond its six sessions, but 16 years later, when I was no longer at the church, the caregiver group was still meeting monthly under the leadership of one of the original group members. The reason this group continued meeting was not only because ongoing group support was very important to the caregiver group, but because one of its members had the necessary leadership skills to continue it. Thus, if you do start a group, it's a good idea to begin developing leadership skills in group members so they can take over the leadership of the group eventually. This enables the group to continue while allowing you to move on to other activities. Helping others develop skills in ministry is an important part of your job and one of the most rewarding.

The shape your practice takes depends on a number of factors such as your own areas of expertise, the nature of the overall faith community ministry, and the size of its staff. What additional nursing specialty knowledge do you bring to this role? Have you worked in acute care, mental health, hospice, home health, or public health? Do you have experience as an educator or administrator? What age groups have you worked with, and which do you enjoy most? It's important to consider these questions so that there is a good fit between you and the faith community in which you'll be working.

If you are hired or placed in a faith community through an institutional program (e.g., hospital or health agency), your areas of expertise and interest will be intentionally matched with a certain faith community's characteristics and health ministry needs. If you work with other FCNs on a volunteer basis, then each of you can do health ministry in areas in which you have the most experience. Of course, even if you've never worked with certain age groups, such as children or older adults, you can always learn to work with them. But initially, your ministry will be easier and more effective if it fits most closely with your individual experience and expertise. To minister effectively and safely in all areas of your practice, assess your learning needs and work to achieve the required competence.

If your faith community has outreach programs such as a homeless ministry or a senior citizen's residence, you may also work with these groups. In these settings, especially, you will often function as a liaison to community resources or as a healthcare advocate, helping people access affordable health care. Ideally, your ministry will involve the whole congregation. This is more likely if the faith community has only a few staff. If the staff is large, you may work primarily with one age group, such as senior citizens. It is not unusual for faith communities to want FCNs to serve this group exclusively because its needs, which often include health concerns, exceed the staff resources of many congregations today. Ministry to this age group involves visiting the homebound, helping them manage chronic health conditions such as diabetes or congestive heart failure, and finding resources for continued independence. The FCN is often seen as the best-equipped staff member to meet these needs.

While the goal of faith community nursing is to increase the health and healing capacity of the entire congregation, it is often more realistic for the FCN to provide direct ministry to specific age groups whose needs are not currently being met by other staff. A particular group may have a need which the faith community perceives can be met best by the FCN ministry. At the same time, the FCN needs to be available to serve everyone.

However, a word of caution: working with only one specific age group may keep you from assisting other members with health concerns and from developing a broad-based health ministry. But if you are free to address other areas of the faith community's health concerns as they arise, this specialized type of faith community nursing practice is just as valid as the one originally envisioned by Rev. Granger Westberg. It may be part of faith community nursing's natural evolution. All

Examples of FCN Functions

- Establish an FCN telephone system. Faith community members can call day or night with a health question and leave a message for the FCN, who answers within 36 hours.

- Provide support to a frightened mother in the morning until she is comfortable giving injected insulin to her newly diagnosed diabetic child.

- Teach the use of a glucometer to senior citizens with arthritis, and monitor the skill until it can be done unassisted.

- Assist adult children on ways to communicate their parents' healthcare needs to doctors.

- Answer questions about medications, and provide guidance on administration (such as the best time to take diuretics to avoid interfering with sleep).

- Contact physicians to clarify medication orders.

- Suggest ways to utilize community health services.

- Instruct parents and teachers on the use of epi pens.

- Assist with writing health protocols for religious and alternative schools.

by Jackie Herzlinger, FCN

developing practices, including nursing itself, change over time. What will not change for faith community nursing is its underlying principle of integrating faith and health through the intentional care of the spirit. In order to do this effectively, you will need to follow the nursing process.

THE NURSING PROCESS

Faith Community Nursing: Scope and Standards of Practice (ANA and HMA 2005) details the actions integral to practicing faith community nursing. Using the nursing process will enable you to address your faith community's specific health concerns in a systematic way and to measure your success. It will also provide a means to communicate what you do to the faith community's staff, health committee, governing body, and membership. Let's look at the standards and explore some ways you can apply them specifically in your work as an FCN.

STANDARD 1. ASSESSMENT

As you begin your wholistic assessment of the faith community, you'll probably be looking at it in a new way. Even if you are practicing in your own faith community, you may not have viewed it from a health perspective. The following questions will help you think about the faith community in this way. What would you say are its major health concerns? What percentage of those in your faith community are retired or are young families? What are the characteristics of the surrounding community, and how do these affect the health of those who live in the area? Where do most of the members live? Has the neighborhood changed since the faith community was established? Try to find answers to these questions when you start your work.

This information will help you know where to begin in addressing health needs and planning health programs. You'll want to learn about the faith community as it is today, but also a little about its history. You may discover some health patterns or learn about demographic and cultural changes that have occurred in it or its surrounding neighborhood that affect health. To get this information, look through the faith community archives and records and talk to people, especially long-time members of the faith community. Ask the senior spiritual leader these questions: What are the most frequent health concerns you see? How many children are born and how many people die each year? This information will give you a beginning sense of the faith community's place in the community and its general health. To better understand the larger health problems in the community, particularly if you're new to an area, contact the local public health department.

A beginning health interest survey of the congregation helps identify the current health issues people are dealing with and what type of health classes they are interested in. You will get the greatest response if you have people complete the survey when they are together as a group. In some faith communities this will be during the main weekly worship service. If allowed, enclose the survey in the worship service bulletin for people to complete and return after worship. You might want to list a variety of health topics for people to choose from, and also have them choose from a list of days and times when they could attend classes. Putting some age group boxes on the sheet for people to check will help you target certain groups. A survey like this also announces the beginning of your ministry and helps people understand your role in the church.

You can collect health information from individuals by having them fill out a health assessment form or by interviewing them. You can create your own assessment form or use a standard guide such as Gordon's Functional Health Patterns (Gordon 2002). The Brief Health Assessment Form that I created can be found in Appendix B. Whatever means you use, you need to be able to collect health data systematically. Taking a full health history the first time you see someone is usually not necessary, nor is it practical. As an FCN, the only time I obtained a comprehensive history at one time was when individuals started a weight management program I'd developed, which included individual health counseling. Otherwise, I gathered information over time as I saw people either in my office, in their homes, or at various faith community activities (and it always surprised me how

> ### Basic Faith Community Assessment Data
> - Number of active members
> - Major health concerns
> - Number of births and deaths annually
> - Demographic makeup (number in each age group, ethnic background, socio-economic status, education level)
> - Environmental hazards
> - Employment level
> - Types of employment
> - Workplace hazards
> - Availability of health care and community resources

many women told me their health concerns in the women's restroom). The FCN must always be sure to protect the confidentiality and privacy of the health or spiritual information provided by a member of the faith community.

Obtaining a health history is just good practice, but for legal reasons, it's especially important before giving health advice. As an FCN, a community social service agency the church supported asked me to check on people in their homes who had recently been ill and/or hospitalized. Since I didn't know the health histories of these people and usually only saw them one time, I decided it would be prudent to primarily assess their needs, encourage them to follow doctor's orders, suggest community resources, and pray with them.

As discussed in Chapter 2, don't forget to include a spiritual assessment as part of the health history (see Appendix A for a Spiritual Assessment Form). Again, you'll have to judge whether it's appropriate for a person to fill out a formal assessment themselves or for you to ask them questions and record the information yourself. A variety of spiritual assessment tools useful for FCN practice are found in the book *Nursing the Spirit* (Wilt and Smucker 2001). A recent spiritual assessment instrument is by Galak, Flannelly, Vane, and Galek (2005).

After you've collected data through assessment and come to some conclusions about a person's health concerns, making a nursing diagnosis will guide your recommendations.

STANDARD 2. DIAGNOSIS

The faith community nurse analyzes the wholistic assessment data to determine the diagnoses or issues. Using a standardized classification (taxonomy) such as the Omaha System (Martin 2005) or nursing diagnoses developed by the North American Nursing Diagnosis Association (NANDA 2004) to label the health issues you've identified will help you organize your care and document it. The Omaha System is a comprehensive practice and documentation tool that includes an assessment component (Problem Classification Scheme), an intervention component (Intervention Scheme), and an outcomes component (Problem Rating Scale for Outcomes). Nursing diagnoses identify actual, perceived, or potential threats to health and personal well-being, as well as a person's response to health conditions or needs. Both systems are recognized by the American Nurses Association.

Nursing diagnosis research is ongoing to refine and improve the system's usefulness. Originally only illness-centered, nursing diagnoses now include wellness diagnoses, which make them more useful to nurses working in health promotion areas such as faith community nursing. Kelley, Frisch, and Avant (1995) developed a trifocal model of nursing diagnoses that conceptualizes the connections between actual, risk, and wellness diagnoses. The model demonstrates the movement toward health and wellness and allows any of NANDA's current diagnostic labels to be used at each of the three levels.

A couple of the FCNs in the program I coordinated used nursing diagnoses and documented them on their monthly report forms using the NANDA numbering system to identify the specific health patterns associated with each diagnosis. This documentation provided a quick and easy way to track predominant health patterns in each nurse's practice. Using some type of classification system will help you more clearly interpret assessment data and determine outcomes and ways to achieve them. Overall, a classification system is a valuable tool for quality practice and documentation which validates and contributes to the development of faith community nursing practice.

Once you've made a nursing diagnosis, share your conclusions with the person or congregation, if possible, to validate your judgment. Then, work together with them to identify desired health outcomes.

STANDARD 3. OUTCOMES IDENTIFICATION

Outcomes terminology may be new to some nurses. It refers to a measure of productivity and accomplishment that healthcare professionals, along with companies and businesses, are being asked to account for and make visible to the public. The faith community nurse identifies expected outcomes for a plan individualized to the patient or the situation.

The Omaha System includes a Problem Rating Scale for Outcomes to measure the knowledge, behavior, and status of clients. It serves as a means to monitor client progress.

The Nursing Outcomes Classification system (NOC) (Moorhead, Johnson, and Maas 2003) is helpful for setting appropriate and realistic outcomes based on nursing diagnoses. Each outcome measure, such as Spiritual Well-Being, is set within a table of associated outcome indicators (e.g., Expression of Faith, Expression of Hope, Prayer), which are on a scale of 1 to 5 (Extremely compromised to Not compromised). This list of indicators (and its associated scale which the nurse marks as a part of assessment) provides the basis of measuring the degree of outcome achievement and helps in identifying the behaviors associated with the outcome, which can guide nursing interventions. (More on outcomes identification is provided in Chapter 9.)

What might be some desired outcomes from a weight management program, for example? Perhaps a person wants to incorporate regular exercise into their weekly schedule or cut down on fats. Other goals may be losing a certain number of pounds, improving overall muscle tone, or lowering cholesterol and blood pressure. Talk with the person to determine outcomes that are desired, appropriate, and realistic. Sometimes it's helpful to break down a long-term outcome into several steps. In this way, a person not only gets a feeling of accomplishment sooner, but you have also documented some interim outcomes, since long-term outcomes may not be evident for some time. Being able to show outcomes over time is especially important for accountability purposes.

For all outcomes, take into consideration the patient's spiritual beliefs and practices, culture, and associated benefits, costs, risks, and current scientific evidence. When you've identified realistic outcomes with the person or group and documented them, you can work to develop a plan to attain them.

Standard 4. Planning

Perhaps the faith community realizes it needs to serve healthier meals or wants to provide health education by holding a health fair. Whatever changes or actions groups or individuals decide on, you'll work with them as they plan, drawing on their personal resources, your support, and other available and appropriate resources in the faith community and the local community. Plans should always include spiritual resources.

If several people in the faith community have similar concerns, you might want to form a support group for them. Also, if someone has recently experienced an illness or crisis but is now physically and emotionally stable and willing to share their experience with others, it may be helpful to match them one-on-one with a person newly experiencing a similar circumstance. Good planning can generate all kinds of such creative health strategies.

As you plan programs to meet the health needs of the congregation, fitting these in with your faith community's overall goals and purposes will better ensure greater participation and success. For instance, if one of the faith community's goals is to increase mission outreach to the surrounding neighborhood, then the FCN might plan and coordinate health screenings or flu immunizations for this group. Also, try to incorporate into your work goals that are common to most faith communities: building a sense of community, enhancing and affirming each person's self-worth, and equipping people to live out their faith.

In planning classes, remember to adapt your teaching strategies to different age groups and styles of learning. Write instructional objectives for your course to guide its preparation and by which to evaluate learning outcomes. Consult a taxonomy of educational objectives for help in writing objectives (Gronlund 1985). As an example, here are some objectives I wrote for the caregivers' support group I developed as an FCN:

1. Describe the emotions experienced by the family in the film "My Mother, My Father."

2. Discuss how the family made decisions about caregiving and living arrangements in the film.

3. Name the community agencies that provide respite care.

4. Describe the purpose and process of estate planning, wills, and power of attorney.

5. Describe the common feelings and behaviors of care receivers.

6. Explain the professional counseling role.

7. Identify ways professional counseling could be helpful to caregivers.

Good planning is essential to successful outcomes. Take time to explore a variety of resources and actions, selecting those that best match the needs and characteristics of the person, congregation, or community.

STANDARD 5. IMPLEMENTATION

Once you and the person or group you're working with has decided on the necessary steps to take in a health plan, you'll support their efforts in many ways: by finding resources, teaching, emotional support, practical assistance, prayer, and frequent contact. As a plan is implemented, you'll frequently reassess the diagnosis, desired outcomes, and make modifications as needed with the person or group involved.

Changing health behaviors is not easy, as we all know when we try to take off those unwanted pounds we've gained over the holidays! First we need to believe it's possible. Next, we decide on an achievable goal and reasonable plan. Can we exercise an hour a day? Having friends to exercise with and encourage, support, and pray for us may make the difference between regaining a normal weight or giving up in defeat.

That one-on-one care and concern nurses are known for is critical in disease prevention and health promotion activities. Faith community nursing is similar to the case management methods that are proving so successful today in health care which closely monitor patients in the community to prevent hospitalization. Accordingly, FCNs contact people whose screening test results are outside the normal range to see if they've followed recommendations. If someone has high blood pressure, you'll want to know if they've seen their doctor or are monitoring their blood pressure regularly. Caring in this way is one of the greatest rewards of faith community nursing. There's nothing more thrilling to an FCN than a person who comes into the office with a big smile to report a lower blood pressure reading and to thank you for helping them to exercise, eat better, and lose weight.

The scope of faith community nursing practice is determined by each state's Nurse Practice Act. However, the health needs of each faith community will determine whether the FCN performs all nursing functions allowed by each state. Some faith communities may want an FCN to give nursing care in a faith-community-based clinic. Advanced practice FCNs, depending on their state laws and federal laws and regulations, are allowed to medically diagnose, order diagnostic tests, and prescribe medications.

Historically, faith community nursing care has not usually included physical care. This self-imposed practice limitation serves to protect and enhance the intentional care of the spirit ministry focus. This comes out of the concern that giving invasive physical care such as flu immunizations, changing dressings, or doing other physical interventions will erode the spiritual component of faith community nursing, making it indistinguishable from home health or hospice nursing. Rather than duplicating these community services, most faith community nurses instead primarily coordinate care by training or supervising others to do these tasks. What if first aid or emergency care is needed? In most cases you'll respond yourself in a crisis. But in order to fulfill the larger purpose of faith community nursing to promote health as wholeness, most FCNs do not regularly provide physical care.

What the FCN is allowed to do may also be restricted by state laws under which other health professionals practice. For instance, when you have lab test results, some state regulations require a physician to read them before you give them to individuals.

STANDARD 6. EVALUATION

All the steps in the nursing process will need to be adapted to working with individuals, groups, or the entire congregation. Thus, evaluation will be done either by assessing one individual's progress toward attainment of outcomes or, alternatively, the overall success of a program or activity, such as a health fair that may also involve the local community.

In the busyness of each day, it's easy to go from one program to the next without evaluating your efforts. But once you make a habit of evaluating, such as at the end of a support group or class series on aging, evaluation becomes second nature. Over time you will appreciate the ways evaluative feedback will improve your work and performance. It's not common for faith community staff to do formal program evaluations, so you may have to make your own forms or find existing forms you can use. A simple evaluation form can be created based on the program objectives you've written by asking if or to what extent these have been met. To get additional feedback, include space on the form for individual written comments or suggestions. Another type of evaluation form that can be used for a variety of programs and one people enjoy filling out has open-ended statements to complete such as, "The most important thing I learned was...," or "I was surprised to learn that...," or "I now think it is possible for me to...."

Your evaluations will also be a way to document the initial outcomes for your interventions. Evaluating your ministry does not have to be a chore or something to fear. Sure, you may get some negative feedback, but overall, people are thoughtful, appreciate your efforts, and are willing to suggest ways to help you improve your developing ministry. Even the negative feedback may ultimately be helpful! Use it to make or recommend process or program changes.

SUMMARY

Faith community nurses function in a variety of ways to integrate faith and health and provide intentional care of the spirit. *Faith Community Nursing: Scope and Standards of Practice* (ANA and HMA 2005) is an important guide to achieving this goal. As you use the nursing process, be sure to include faith elements and resources, always keeping in mind that you are practicing within the beliefs and values of a particular faith community. Faith community nursing challenges you to be creative. Don't be afraid to ask for help or share ideas with others. By working with faith community and local community groups, multiple resources will help you better meet the varied health needs of the faith community. Shape your practice to your faith community's health needs. Continually evaluate your ministry. Involve your health committee and the pastoral staff in developing your role.

REFERENCES AND RESOURCES

All online references and resources were current September 30, 2008.

REFERENCES

American Nurses Association and Health Ministries Association. 2005. *Faith community nursing: Scope and standards of practice.* Silver Spring, MD: Nursesbooks.org.

Daehling, E., and K. Soder-Alderfer, eds. 1984. *Ministries of healing.* Philadelphia: Parish Life Press.

Galek, K., K. Flannelly, A. Vane, and R. Galek. 2005. Assessing a patient's spiritual needs: A comprehensive instrument. *Holistic Nursing Practice* 19 (2): 62–69.

Gordon, M. 2002. *Manual of nursing diagnosis.* St. Louis: C.V. Mosby.

Gronlund, N. 1985. *Stating objectives for classroom instruction,* 2nd ed. New York: Macmillan.

Kelley, J., N. Frisch, and K. Avant. 1995 A trifocal model of nursing diagnosis: Wellness reinforced. *Nursing Diagnosis* 6 (3): 123–28.

Larson, D., J. Swyers, and M. McCullough. 1998. *Scientific research on spirituality and health: A consensus report.* Rockville, MD: National Institute for Healthcare Research.

Martin, K. 2005. *The Omaha system: A key to practice, documentation, and information management,* 2nd ed. St. Louis: Elsevier.

Moorhead, S., M. Johnson, and M. Maas, eds. 2003. *Nursing outcomes classification (NOC,* 3rd ed. St. Louis: Mosby.

North American Nursing Diagnosis Association (NANDA). 2004. *Nursing diagnoses: Definitions and classification 2005–2006.* NANDA.

Tubesing, N., and D. Tubesing, eds. 1986/1994. *Structured exercises in wellness promotion,* vol. 4. Duluth, MN: Whole Person Associates.

Tubesing, D., and N. Tubesing. 1991. *Seeking your healthy balance.* Duluth, MN: Whole Person Associates.

Westberg, G. 1987. *The parish nurse.* Park Ridge, IL: Parish Nurse Resource Center.

Wilt, D., and C. Smucker. 2001. *Nursing the spirit.* Washington, DC: American Nurses Publishing.

SUGGESTED RESOURCES

Adams, G., R. Hampton, T. Gullotta, R. Weissberg, and B. Ryan, eds. 1997. *Enhancing children's wellness.* Thousand Oaks, CA: Sage.

American Nurses Association. 2001. *Code of ethics for nurses with interpretive statements.* Washington, DC: American Nurses Publishing.

American Nurses Association. 2005. *Principles for documentation* (brochure). Washington, DC: ANA.

Benson, H., and E. Stuart. 1992. *The wellness book.* New York: Simon and Schuster.

Buehler, D., and R. Tiemeyer, eds. 1985. *Health and healing in the Bible.* Philadelphia: Parish Life Press.

Chase-Ziolek, M. 2005. *Health, healing, and wholeness: Engaging congregations in ministries of health.* Cleveland, OH: Pilgrim.

Clark, C. 2003. *Group leadership skills.* New York: Springer.

Clark, C., ed. 2001. *Health promotion in communities: Holistic and wellness approaches.* New York: Springer.

Clark, C. 1996. *Wellness practitioner: Concepts, research, and strategies,* 2nd ed. New York: Springer.

Cloud, H., and J. Townsend. 2003. *Leading small groups that help people grow.* Grand Rapids, MI: Zondervan.

Coenen, A., D. Weis, M. Schank, and R. Matheus. 1999. Describing parish nurse practice using the nursing minimum data set. *Public Health Nursing* 16 (6): 412–16.

Condon, M. 2002. *Women's health: Body, mind, spirit, an integrated approach to wellness and illness.* Upper Saddle River, NJ: Prentice Hall.

Dochterman, J., and G. Bulechek, eds. 2003. *Nursing interventions classification (NIC),* 4th ed. St. Louis: Mosby.

Dochterman, J., and D. Jones, eds. 2003. *Unifying nursing languages: The harmonization of NANDA, NIC, and NOC.* Washington, DC: American Nurses Publishing.

Doenges, M., M. Moorhouse, and A. Geissler-Murr. 2002. *Nurse's pocket guide: Diagnoses, interventions, and rationales,* 8th ed. Philadelphia: F.A. Davis.

Dossey, L. 1993. *Healing words: The power of prayer and the practice of medicine.* San Francisco: Harper.

Egan, G. 2001. *The skilled helper: A problem-management and opportunity-development approach to helping,* 7th ed. Belmont, CA: Wadsworth.

Fite, R. 1999. The congregation as a workplace. In A.Solari-Twadell and M. McDermott, eds., *Parish nursing: Promoting whole person health within faith communities,* pp. 123–33. Thousand Oaks, CA: Sage.

Frisch, N., B. Dossey, C. Guzzeta, and J. Quinn. 2000. *AHNA standards of holistic nursing practice: Guidelines for caring and healing.* Gaithersburg, MD: Aspen.

George, C., W. Gird, and R. Coleman. 2001. *Nine keys to effective small group leadership: How lay leaders can establish dynamic and healthy small cells, classes, or teams.* Berkeley, CA: Kingdom.

Gillis, A. 1995. Exploring nursing outcomes for health promotion. *Nursing Forum* 30 (2): 5–12.

Gordon, M. 1994. *Nursing diagnosis: Process and application,* 3rd ed. St. Louis: Mosby.

Guarneri, M. 2006. *The heart speaks: A cardiologist reveals the secret language of healing.* New York: Touchstone.

Guzzetta, C. E., et al. 1989. *Clinical assessment tools for use with nursing diagnoses.* St. Louis: Mosby Year Book.

Hale, W., and H. Koenig. 2003. *Healing bodies and souls: A practical guide for congregations.* Minneapolis, MN: Augsburg Fortress.

Hankinson, S., G. Colditz, J. Manson, and F. Speizer, eds. 2001. *Healthy women, healthy lives.* New York: Simon and Schuster Source.

Hickman, J. 2006. *Faith community nursing.* Philadelphia, PA: Lippincott Williams and Wilkins.

Hughes, C., J. Trofino, B. O'Brien, J. Mack, and M. Marrinau. 2001. Primary care parish nursing: Outcomes and implications. *Nursing Administration Quarterly* 26 (1): 45–59.

Johnson, M., G. Bulechek, J. Dochterman, M. Maas, and S. Moorhead. 2001. *Nursing diagnoses, outcomes, and interventions: NANDA, NIC, and NOC linkages.* St. Louis: Mosby. (2003: also available in CD-ROM from Mosby.)

Koenig, H. 2006. *Faith and mental health.* West Conshohocken, PA: Templeton Foundation.

Koenig, H., and H. Cohen, eds. 2002. *The link between religion and health: PNI and the faith factor.* Oxford: Oxford University Press.

Matthews, D. 1998. *The faith factor.* New York: Viking.

McBride, N. 1998. *Real small groups just don't happen: Nurturing relationships in your small group.* Colorado Springs, CO: Navpress.

McCloskey, J., and G. Bulechek, eds. 2000. *Nursing interventions classification (NIC),* 3rd ed. St. Louis: Mosby.

Miller, C. 2003. *Nursing for wellness in older adults: Theory and practice.* Philadelphia, PA: Lippincott Williams and Wilkins.

Miller, L. 2004. *Faith and health: A framework for Christian nurses.* Victoria, BC: Trafford.

Moberg, D. 2001. *Aging and spirituality: Spiritual dimensions of aging theory, research, practice and policy.* New York: Haworth.

Morris, E. 2001. The relationship of spirituality to coronary heart disease. *Alternative Therapies in Health and Medicine* 7 (5): 96–98.

Nardi, D., J. Petr, and R. Meade, eds. 2002. *Community health and wellness assessment: A step by step guide.* Albany, NY: Delmar.

Nelson, G. 1999. Pastoral reflections. In A. Solari-Twadell and M. McDermott , eds., *Parish nursing: Promoting whole person health within faith communities,* pp. 161–67. Thousand Oaks, CA: Sage.

O'Connor, C. 2001. Characteristics of spiritual assessment and prayer in holistic nursing. *Nursing Clinics of North America* 36(1): 33-46.

Paloma, M. 1993. The effects of prayer on mental well-being. *Second Opinion* 18 (3): 37–51.

Prakash, D. 1989. *Health and medicine in the Hindu tradition: Continuity and cohesion.* New York: Crossroad/Herder and Herder.

Pravikoff, D., S. Pierce, and A. Tanner. 2003. Are nurses ready for evidence-based practice? *American Journal of Nursing* 103 (5): 95–96.

Rahman, F. 1998. *Health and medicine in the Islamic tradition: Change and identity.* Lahore, Pakistan: Kazi.

Ray, O. 2004. How the mind hurts and heals the body. *American Psychologist* 59 (1): 1–12.

Stolte, K. 1996. *Wellness: Nursing diagnosis for health promotion.* Philadelphia, PA: Lippincott Williams and Wilkins.

Swinney, J., C. Anson-Wonkka, E. Maki, and J. Corneau. 2001. Community assessment: A church community and the parish nurse. *Public Health Nursing* 18 (1): 40–44.

Thomas, D., and M. King. 2000. Parish nursing assessment—What should you know? *Home Healthcare Nurse Manager* 4 (5): 11–13.

Thomas, S., and H. Pollio. 2002. *Listening to patients: A phenomenological approach to nursing research and practice.* New York: Springer.

VandeCreek, L. 1999. *Spiritual care for persons with dementia.* New York: Haworth.

Waltz, C., and O. Strickland, eds. 1991. *Measurement of nursing outcomes: Measuring client self-care and coping skills.* New York: Springer.

Watson, J. 1988. *Nursing: Human science and human care.* New York: National League for Nursing.

Weis, D., M. Schank, A. Coenen, and R. Matheus. 2002. Parish nurse practice with client aggregates. *Journal of Community Health Nursing* 19 (2): 105–113.

Westberg, G. 1979. *Theological roots of wholistic health care.* Hinsdale, IL: Wholistic Health Centers, Inc.

Wilkinson, J. 1999. *Nursing diagnosis handbook with NIC interventions and NOC outcomes,* 7th ed. Upper Saddle River, NJ: Prentice Hall.

Worthington, E. 2006. *The power of forgiving.* West Conshohocken, PA: Templeton Foundation.

ORGANIZATIONAL RESOURCES: NURSING

Center for Nursing Classification and Clinical Effectiveness (NIC, NOC), University of Iowa: **www.nursing.uiowa.edu/cnc**

University of Kansas' The Community Tool Box, which provides over 6,000 pages of practical information to support work in promoting community health and development: **www.ctb.ukans.edu**

Duke University's Center for the Study of Religion/Spirituality and Health: **garcia.geri.duke.edu/religion/index.html.** Research News and Opportunities in Science and Theology (monthly newspaper): **www.researchnewsonline.org**

International Journal of Nursing Terminologies and Classifications: **www.blackwellpublishing.com/journal.asp?ref=1541-5147**

NANDA–International Nursing Journal: National Center for Complementary and Alternative Medicine (NCCAM): **www.nccam.nih.gov**

North American Nursing Diagnosis Association International (NANDA-International): (www.nanda.org). *International Journal of Nursing Terminologies and Classification*: **www.blackwellpublishing.com/journal.asp?ref=1541-5147**

ORGANIZATIONAL RESOURCES: CHRISTIAN DENOMINATIONAL HEALTH MINISTRY INFORMATION

The Evangelical Lutheran Church in America: **www.elca.org/dcs/healthmin.html**

The Episcopal Church, USA: **www.episcopalhealthministries.org/links.html**

The Presbyterian Church, USA: **www.pcusa.org/health/usa/parishnursing/taskforce.htm**

Research News and Opportunities in Science and Theology (monthly newspaper): **www.researchnewsonline.org**

United Methodist Church: **gbgm-umc.org/health/congmin**

CHAPTER 5

PRACTICING PROFESSIONALLY: STANDARDS OF PROFESSIONAL PERFORMANCE

The longer we practice, the more we need standards of professional performance. The more changes that take place in health care, the greater the need and challenge to increase our skills and knowledge through continuing education and research to maintain a quality practice. Faith community nursing will continue to adapt to changing demographics, disease patterns, national emergencies, and healthcare delivery models. Ongoing collaboration with healthcare colleagues and evaluation of our work is essential to meeting our nation's healthcare needs. Wise use of our resources and appropriate response to emerging environmental threats are required by FCNs as nursing leaders. New healthcare technology will continue to challenge FCNs in caring for people. FCNs will be involved in the faith community response to the many ethical issues challenging faith communities today. Following these standards is increasingly necessary in our fast-changing world.

STANDARD 7. QUALITY OF PRACTICE

The faith community nurse systematically enhances the quality and effectiveness of faith community nursing practice. This involves continually monitoring, evaluating, and incorporating new knowledge to initiate changes in faith community nursing practice for desired outcomes. Quality assurance programs were mandated for hospitals in the early 1970s by the Joint Commission on Accreditation of Healthcare Organizations. Evidence of Japan's business success in the 1950s and a desire to be more competitive in the world market led American companies to incorporate Dr. W. Edwards Deming's (an American statistician) ideas for achieving quality. Since then, all types of businesses and organizations have adopted aspects of what was originally an industrial management idea. Perhaps you've helped write a vision statement, been a member of a quality circle, redesigned jobs, or put into practice a self-managing team, all techniques rooted in Deming's ideas.

Which of these quality assurance measures will be used by the faith community will depend on its needs and experience with such measures. You may be able to help the staff incorporate some of these measures into faith community work. Your adherence, however, to the Faith Community Nursing Standards of Practice and Standards of Professional Performance will be the basis of quality in your practice.

Standards of Professional Performance

- Quality of Practice
- Education
- Professional Practice Evaluation
- Collegiality
- Collaboration
- Ethics
- Research
- Resource Utilization
- Leadership

(ANA and HMA 2005, page x.)

STANDARD 8. EDUCATION

The faith community nurse attains knowledge and competency that reflects current nursing practice. Before many faith community nursing preparation courses were available, nurses learned about faith community nursing on their own from Rev. Granger Westburg's writings or from practicing FCNs. Today, numerous faith community nursing courses are available throughout the country, some of which use the Parish Nurse Core Curriculum developed and sponsored by the IPNRC. Books and manuals on faith community nursing continue to proliferate but are no substitute for formal education programs. To ensure a quality practice, you need to take some type of preparation course. To find courses, contact the IPNRC and HMA, or check the Internet. Online courses are being offered for nurses who do not have a course available in their location.

When you begin faith community nursing, you are probably transitioning from another nursing practice area. While you will be current on the latest information on diseases and treatments in that area, you may need to broaden your knowledge beyond that area for the FCN role. And over time, unless you also practice in a healthcare facility and are intentional about keeping up with nursing and healthcare advances, your knowledge base may gradually become outdated.

A good way to obtain continuing education is through workshops, especially those offered at annual nursing conferences. Continuing education is only one of the many benefits of belonging to professional organizations, such as the American Nurses Association. The Health Ministries Association, which is the FCN's professional specialty organization, and the International Parish Nurse Resource Center also offer annual conferences, which provide excellent educational opportunities for learning more about faith community nursing as well as provide spiritual nourishment and networking opportunities.

In addition, as discussed earlier, you'll need to learn spiritual care skills and continue to develop your personal faith. Take time to read and study religious literature, go to spiritual workshops and retreats, and practice daily spiritual disciplines, such as prayer or meditation. From personal experience, I guarantee that the rewards of this ongoing spiritual development will enhance your practice and personal life.

STANDARD 9. PROFESSIONAL PRACTICE EVALUATION

The faith community nurse evaluates his or her own nursing practice in relation to professional practice standards and guidelines, relevant statutes, rules, and regulations.

Take time to evaluate your performance regularly. Answering the following questions will help you evaluate your work:

- What have my priorities been this year? Do these represent the congregation's assessed health needs? Am I following the Health Committee's priorities? Why or why not?

- What programs have been successful this year and which have not? What are the reasons for this? What do I need to change to make some more successful?

- What new health needs have arisen this year? How will I address these?

- What problems or barriers have I encountered this year? What will I do about them?

- What did I learn from my mistakes this year?

- How is the "fit" between my ministry and the faith community's?

- How are my relationships with the staff? With the faith community? With community agencies?

Plan to meet annually for a performance evaluation with your supervisor or whoever does faith community staff evaluations. If you are not a part of an institutional program, you may have to be the one to initiate an annual review. If an evaluation form is not provided, find or create one that can be filled out both by yourself and your supervisor. This facilitates discussion and provides two perspectives on your strengths as well as areas needing improvement. Others may be more objective about your work and are often more positive about it than you are. Many of us tend to be excessively critical of ourselves and our work.

Hopefully you will receive supervisory feedback, not only at an annual evaluation but throughout the year. That is why it is so important to meet regularly (weekly, if possible) with your supervisor. The formal year-end review should be only a part of the overall evaluation process. Both of you should work to develop a way to communicate effectively and efficiently so that the annual review will be something you look forward to and find a valuable help in improving your work.

Standard 10. Collegiality

The faith community nurse interacts with and contributes to the professional development of peers and colleagues. As you continue to educate yourself for faith community nursing, be willing to share what you learn with other FCNs and health ministry colleagues. Meet with other FCNs, if possible, to learn from each other's successes and mistakes. If you don't have a peer FCN group available through a hospital or health agency, you can form a group in your community with like-minded individuals or a Health Ministries Association chapter (HMA) (see resources at the end of chapter). Much of my own faith community nursing expertise evolved through membership in HMA, attending and presenting at the IPNRC's annual Westberg Symposium, and through meeting with a regional Parish Nurse Program Coordinators' Group.

Another way to share your expertise is to serve as a community health preceptor for nursing students. Contact the community health nursing faculty of colleges or universities near you to volunteer. With the shift to more community-based health care, there is an increasing need for community health clinical sites for students.

Faith Community Nurse and Community Collaboration Ideas

- Community health fair
- Bicycle safety training
- Sexual abstinence program
- Public health department community projects
- Police department home safety inspections
- Health screenings
- Flu immunization program

STANDARD 11. COLLABORATION

Collaboration involves working together with the patient, spiritual leaders, members of the faith community, and local community. I've mentioned before the importance of combining your efforts with those of others in your community on health promotion and disease prevention ventures, such as the annual flu immunization programs, which most communities have each fall. Faith communities often serve as immunization sites, and FCNs can coordinate these efforts. Find out what is going on in your community in disease prevention, and get included in these efforts. Through collaboration, everyone's efforts can be multiplied. Collaboration has been the basis of our government's ongoing efforts to financially support local faith programs, which are having many positive effects on community health. This is most recently evident in the efforts of cleaning up and rebuilding in the Gulf area after Hurricane Katrina.

Of course, you'll also collaborate with your client (faith community member, faith community, community) and seek out knowledgeable individuals (spiritual leader, faith community staff, healthcare and other professionals) to help you in your ministry. In addition to improving your ability to help your client or community, forming these relationships can keep you from feeling alone in your work. In all types of ministry, including faith community nursing, a person can feel as though he or she is working alone. Because you will not be coming into contact with other professionals as you would in a healthcare setting, you will have to make an effort to collaborate. When face-to-face meetings are impractical, use the phone and e-mail to share information and learn from others.

Sometimes a person's situation is beyond your expertise and you'll need to know whom to refer that person to. When you refer, you'll need to be aware of and follow the current federal patient privacy rules for protection of medical records, which came out of the Health Insurance Portability and Accountability Act of 1996 (HIPAA). In general, these rules require that healthcare providers limit the disclosure of personal health information to the *minimum necessary* to achieve a given purpose. For a more complete explanation of the standards to protect the privacy of personal health information, see the U.S. Department of Health and Human Services Web site: www.hhs.gov/ocr/hipaa.

STANDARD 12. ETHICS

The faith community nurse integrates ethical provisions in all areas of practice. Ethics involves what is right and best in practice. FCNs follow nursing's ethics as delineated in *Code of Ethics for Nurses with Interpretive Statements* (ANA 2001; see also pg. 60). At the heart of ethical behavior is a professional and therapeutic client–nurse relationship. It follows that the FCN respects clients, is nonjudgmental, nondiscriminatory, and maintains confidentiality.

Many ethical healthcare issues can involve FCNs. For example, you may be asked to help people understand end-of-life issues and guide them to make decisions about medical treatment consistent with their spiritual beliefs. You may also be asked to serve as someone's healthcare advocate. Your ability to define medical terms, describe treatments, and relate to healthcare professionals on someone's behalf is invaluable to people unfamiliar with these things.

Confidentiality is an important ethical standard. Not only will you ensure privacy by meeting with people in a private space, you must also uphold their right to privacy by acting in accord with the most recent federal healthcare privacy rules (HIPAA).

When I asked my own faith community's FCN, Rachel Hallam, what she thought would be most important to include in this handbook, she said:

> It is imperative that an FCN keep the confidentiality of those who speak with her or him. I think that it is even more difficult to do this in a faith community setting because everyone knows everyone and will ask, "What is so and so's problem?" or "How is so and so doing?" It is hard to give out some information without giving out too much. I think it is a must that the FCN be very careful not to make offhand remarks to others who might figure out who the FCN is referring to. Confidentiality is a much bigger issue in a faith community setting than it ever was in the hospital setting. I feel like I am on a tightrope sometimes when it comes to how much to reveal [to the spiritual leader] about the people that I visit.

Hold everything people tell you in confidence and protect their health records. Before you share confidential information with the staff, ask a person's permission to do so. The only exception to this is in cases where a person is likely to harm him- or herself or others or in an abuse situation where professional mandatory reporting is required.

Be aware that other government healthcare regulations (such as infection control, disease reporting, and mandatory abuse reporting) and institutional credentialing reviews may also apply to faith community nursing, especially if your practice is sponsored by a healthcare institution.

Typical Ethical Healthcare Situations

Faith community nurses can give wise counsel in the following situations:
- Advance directives
- Resuscitative measures
- Discontinuing life support
- Beginning artificial feeding
- Pregnancy concerns
- Organ donation
- Treatment concerns (possible conflict with religious beliefs)

STANDARD 13. RESEARCH

The faith community nurse integrates research findings into practice. Part of your ongoing education is paying attention to nursing and other health-related research that is relevant to faith community nursing. Regularly read professional nursing journals as well as other journals relevant to faith community nursing, such as *The Journal of Pastoral Care* (www.jpcp.org). The nursing profession advocates evidence-based practice, which is practice that is research based. As you read research articles and consider implementing the results in your practice, but are unsure of the quality of the research, consult someone who has research knowledge or experience in that area of practice.

Because research is the basis for improving nursing practice, you will want to support research in any way you can. Although it can be time-consuming, it is exciting and rewarding to be a part of a research study, especially one on faith community nursing. The

THE CODE OF ETHICS FOR NURSES

1. The nurse, in all professional relationships, practices with compassion and respect for the inherent dignity, worth, and uniqueness of every individual, unrestricted by considerations of social or economic status, personal attributes, or the nature of health problems.

2. The nurse's primary commitment is to the patient, whether an individual, family, group, or community.

3. The nurse promotes, advocates for, and strives to protect the health, safety, and rights of the patient.

4. The nurse is responsible and accountable for individual nursing practice and determines the appropriate delegation of tasks consistent with the nurse's obligation to provide optimum patient care.

5. The nurse owes the same duties to self as to others, including the responsibility to preserve integrity and safety, to maintain competence, and to continue personal and professional growth.

6. The nurse participates in establishing, maintaining, and improving healthcare environments and conditions of employment conducive to the provision of quality health care and consistent with the values of the profession through individual and collective action.

7. The nurse participates in the advancement of the profession through contributions to practice, education, administration, and knowledge development.

8. The nurse collaborates with other health professionals and the public in promoting community, national, and international efforts to meet health needs.

9. The profession of nursing, as represented by associations and their members, is responsible for articulating nursing values, for maintaining the integrity of the profession and its practice, and for shaping social policy.

(ANA 2001, p. 4)

results of a study done on our program validated our experience of the value of faith community nursing to our community (Wallace, Tuck, Boland, and Witucki 2002). Nursing researchers, such as the University of Iowa NOC group, seek input from FCNs especially regarding spiritual interventions and outcomes. Since most people are unfamiliar with faith community nursing and what FCNs have to offer in the development of nursing knowledge, you may have to take the initiative to be involved in research. Whenever possible, introduce yourself to researchers working in your area of interest, and volunteer to work with them in some way on their project. They may want to interview you or people you care for in the congregation. You can help the researchers gain access to the faith community by helping the staff and members understand the purpose of the research and what would be required of them to take part.

STANDARD 14. RESOURCE UTILIZATION

The faith community nurse considers factors related to safety, effectiveness, cost, and impact on practice in the planning and delivery of nursing services. As you help your client access community resources, you'll want to consider these aspects of resource utilization. You'll select those that are most appropriate, accessible, acceptable, and affordable to each person. You may provide the person with a list of resources to choose from. In some cases, the person may want you to select the resource and make the contact. Not only will the client's beliefs and values (such as sexual abstinence programs versus instruction on the use of protective devices, such as condoms) direct the faith community nurse to certain resources, but the faith community's position on certain social issues will as well. In some health situations, such as an unintended pregnancy, the FCN will want to suggest resources that are congruent with the faith community's beliefs. Abortion, for example, is one area the FCN should discuss with the senior spiritual leaders before the FCN starts work in a faith community.

When a client you're seeing has a financial need related to a health issue, ask if the faith community has some discretionary funds to help people that the FCN may access. Most FCNs have few, if any, financial resources budgeted to them initially for these purposes. This may change as your ministry develops and you make needs known.

STANDARD 15. LEADERSHIP

The leadership role and responsibilities of the faith community nurse are discussed in the next chapter (Chapter 6).

SUMMARY

The Standards of Professional Performance are particularly important in helping to shape and develop a new nursing specialty such as faith community nursing. They serve to guide the FCN in establishing and maintaining a quality practice. The time spent putting these standards into practice provides many opportunities to review program goals and objectives, order priorities, evaluate results, improve performance, and plan for the future.

REFERENCES AND RESOURCES

All online references and resources were current September 30, 2008.

REFERENCES

American Nurses Association (ANA). 2001. *Code of ethics for nurses with interpretive statements.* Washington, DC: American Nurses Publishing.

American Nurses Association (ANA) and Health Ministries Association (HMA). 2005. *Faith community nursing: Scope and standards of practice.* Silver Spring, MD: Nursesbooks.org.

Wallace, D., I. Tuck, C. Boland, and J. Witucki. 2002. Client perceptions of parish nursing. *Public Health Nursing* 19 (2): 128–35.

SUGGESTED RESOURCES

Basler, B. 2003. Your eyes only—mostly. *AARP Bulletin* 44 (7): 20.

Guzzeta, C. 2000. Holistic nursing research. In B. Dossey, et al., eds., *Holistic nursing: A handbook for practice,* 3rd ed., pp. 187–202. Gaithersburg, MD: Aspen.

Norlander, L. 2001. *To comfort always: A nurse's guide to end-of-life care.* Washington, DC: American Nurses Publishing.

Pacquiao, D. 2003. Cultural competence in ethical decision making. In M. Andrews and J. Boyle, eds., *Transcultural concepts in nursing care,* pp. 503–532. Philadelphia: Lippincott Williams and Wilkins.

Weis, D., M. Schank, and R. Matheus. 2006. The process of empowerment: A parish nurse perspective. *Journal of Holistic Nursing* 24 (1): 17–24.

ORGANIZATIONAL RESOURCES

The Health Privacy Project offers information of privacy rights and protections: **www.healthprivacy.org**.

HIPAA, U.S. Department of Health and Human Services: **www.hhs.gov/ocr/hipaa**

ADDITIONAL RESOURCES

Journal of Pastoral Care: **www.jpcp.org**

CHAPTER 6

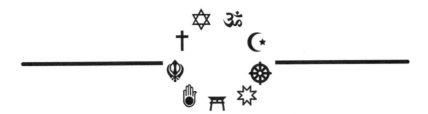

YOU DON'T HAVE TO DO IT ALL YOURSELF: BEING A LEADER

My work as an FCN was divided between caring for the congregation and providing services to the surrounding neighborhood. In addition to working with two inner-city community agencies, I also joined efforts with the Catholic community workers who lived in the area. In talking with them about the health needs of the neighborhood children, they suggested we hold a children's health fair in the faith community building. They would recruit the children and provide transportation, and I would organize the fair.

The church was happy to host the fair, but I knew I couldn't do it all myself. I already had several members who were nurses helping me take monthly blood pressure readings. I talked with them and several volunteered to help with the fair. I selected some Red Cross educational materials to use, met with the nurses to plan, and asked some other faith community members to handle the snack time. With everyone working together, the event was a success. None of us could have accomplished as much by ourselves.

As an FCN, you are the leader of health ministry in the faith community. You will help people learn about wholistic health by making it visible through teaching, counseling, visitation, and spiritual care. As a leader you will guide and direct others as they work toward greater health and wholeness and assist you with this ministry.

STANDARD 15. LEADERSHIP

While being a member of the faith community staff automatically places you in a leadership role, you may not be able to immediately assume that role because faith community nursing is a new role for you and there is so much to learn. But it won't take long for you to get acquainted and feel confident in leading the faith community in health ministry activities. You'll build on the leadership experience you already have from your previous nursing work and from working in your own faith community or with community organizations.

As a leader you'll work to inspire, motivate, and enable others to work together. One of the hallmarks of faith communities is the way people care for each other. They provide practical, emotional, and spiritual support by taking meals to the homebound, driving someone to a doctor's appointment, listening, and praying with someone. FCN Jackie Herzlinger says this about her practice of Jewish congregational nursing: "Congregational nursing is about the ongoing transformation of the faith community into a source of health and healing for all its members." As you go about your work, stay alert for opportunities to connect people to one another in these ways. Often you will see a need that someone in the faith community can meet. In this way the FCN acts as a coordinator of care, bridging members' needs to resources and to each other. FCN Vonda Jennings gives an example from her practice.

> Recently I was working in my office when the phone rang. I answered and a distressed lady told me her story. Her name was Amy. She said she had called all over town looking for a piece of equipment and something just told her to call the church. She shared how her father had cancer and her mother could no longer lift him to provide care. I asked her to tell me what she needed. She replied that she needed a lift chair. I sat speechless. A few weeks earlier, a young couple within our congregation had told me that they had a lift chair they would like to pass on to someone in need. I had told them I would be in touch, and that very morning I had called about the lift chair. I told the lady that I would find someone to pick it up that week. Fifteen minutes after I called about the lift chair, I received the call from Amy. I told Amy that God had already answered her prayer. I passed on the information needed about the chair and hung up the phone. At that moment, I saw God use my role in faith community nursing to do what he does best—miracles!

Many faith communities have ways to learn about their members' talents and willingness to serve. In my faith community we fill out what are called Time and Talent cards each year. If the faith community gathers this type of information, it can help you match the abilities of one member to the needs of another.

As members become involved in your health ministry activities, they will increasingly see it as an integral part of the faith community's overall ministry and take ownership of it. It's tempting, and sometimes easier, to just do things yourself, especially when you're new and don't know many people. But that is one of the main reasons you should ask people to help you. You need people to connect you with others. One of the first groups to invite to be part of your work is your health committee.

WORKING WITH YOUR HEALTH COMMITTEE

The health committee was Rev. Granger Westburg's idea and has proven to be a very wise one. The people on your health committee agree to serve in this way because they are interested in helping you establish and develop a health ministry for their faith community.

Whenever possible, involve them in what you are doing, whether it is in planning, prioritizing, or hands-on help teaching a class, leading a support group, or helping with a health fair.

Initially, a separate health committee is better able to give the time and attention needed to establish your ministry. To help retain members, consider setting up a rotation membership schedule. For example, have one-third of the committee rotate off each year and new members join for a three-year period of service. After faith community nursing has become firmly established, the faith community may choose to discontinue the health committee. If this happens, it is important to find another committee to work with whose work fits well with your own.

Leadership Principles

- You don't have to do it all yourself. Ask for help.
- Inspire, motivate, and enable others to help you develop the faith community's health ministry.
- Form a health committee and involve it in your work.
- Provide volunteer training and ongoing support.
- Remember to thank volunteers.
- Be a bridge connecting members in ministry to each other.
- Be a team player: Help other staff succeed in ministry. See that your work contributes to the faith community's overall goals.

WORKING WITH YOUR FCN VOLUNTEERS

I believe how you relate to people you work with is central to being a successful leader. This is especially important because the faith community is primarily a volunteer organization. The people you work with give their time freely on top of their regular work hours. Thus, the time they give to the faith community is necessarily limited. For these reasons you'll want to make their volunteer experience a rewarding one.

You probably know what it's like to be a volunteer. Your experience as a volunteer may have been very rewarding or rather disappointing. Thinking back to these experiences, what made the difference between them? If it was a good experience, you most likely did something you were interested in, had some ability for, and felt appreciated. A bad experience might have been a job you were not well prepared for and found stressful. Or perhaps no one ever thanked you for what you did and you felt stuck in the position with no way to quit gracefully.

You've probably heard of the Three R's of working with volunteers: Recruitment, Retention, and Recognition. They're easy to remember and easy to do. First you'll find people to help you who interested in what you're doing. Then you need to tell them about the job. To help you do this, you can create a simple job description. This will let the person know the job requirements exactly. If either you or the person volunteering thinks the job is not a good match, acknowledging that at this point helps to prevent future problems. Recruiting volunteers will get easier as you get to know more people and learn about their interests and abilities.

Once you have volunteers, you'll want to retain them. You may need to provide some initial training, such as orienting nurses who will help you with blood-pressure screening. For example, you may need to introduce them to the recording form and guidelines you'll be using in giving recommendations for follow-up care. In addition to training, provide any material resources needed to do the job.

Lay caregiving training programs, such as the BeFriender Program or Stephen Ministry, both Christian-oriented programs, are excellent ways to develop lay ministry skills. These programs include training in communication, spiritual care, short-term crisis counseling, and ways to maintain confidentiality. Such programs may already exist in the faith community, or you may be asked to help begin one. Once developed, the trained people provide an excellent source of volunteers to help meet the ministry and health needs the FCN identifies.

As you work with your volunteers, an attitude of appreciation, encouragement, and support will build friendships between you that will make the experience mutually enjoyable. If a person has a good volunteer experience, he or she is more likely to volunteer another time. One of my friends who volunteers at a local arts organization tells me that no one wants to work with the new director there because of the demeaning way she treats volunteers. How you treat people will affect your ability to recruit and retain volunteers.

Receiving recognition and appreciation for paid work is important, but it is even more important to an unpaid volunteer. There are many ways you can thank your volunteers. A simple verbal or written thank you may be all that's needed. If you have a large number of people helping you throughout the year, you might want to have some kind of annual volunteer celebration to include everyone. Depending on your budget, you could give small gifts or award personalized certificates, which you can buy pre-made or design and print yourself on a computer. If you've ever received this type of recognition, you know how much these small tokens of appreciation mean.

Involving the faith community in your work will keep you from getting burned out on ministry and enable you to get to know more people in the faith community sooner. Being a leader involves not only being a knowledgeable professional who is enthusiastic and personable but one who provides the necessary encouragement and support to those who volunteer to help. FCN Vonda Jennings relates this example of the difference she and volunteers made in someone's life:

> There is a senior living facility next door to our church that we adopted to assist in various ways. We have held Bible studies, prepared parties, and provided meals for the residents there. One day I received a call from the manager that one of the residents who lived alone with no family assistance needed his apartment cleaned. If he did not get his apartment cleaned he would be evicted, a rule of this government-supported housing. He had never let anyone into his apartment before. He also had a reputation of harassing women.
>
> I accepted the job and began to pray that I could find the volunteers that I needed. The two volunteers and I met and went to the apartment. We met the man, and upon entering his apartment it was obvious it needed a lot of cleaning. The ladies asked, "Where do we start?" I simply stated, "We start with prayer." We held hands and prayed that morning for Mr. Arp and that God would abide in his home. We worked for hours, but left that home looking spic and span. We provided dinner that night for Mr. Arp, also. We left exhausted but glorifying God for the joy we felt in our hearts.
>
> After that day, Mr. Arp became more cooperative with the management. He took part in the men's Bible study and was open to talking about his faith. We were told he was a changed man. Mr. Arp became very ill a few months later and passed away after a sudden illness. I visited him as he was dying and shared my faith with him.

Helping Mr. Arp was a meaningful experience for all of us, and I believe Mr. Arp was changed by our kindness. We felt God move into that home that morning and I believe He never left.

THE MINISTRY TEAM

In recent years, the emphasis in organizations and companies has been on developing work teams. Employees are trained in small groups to learn ways to use each other's ideas and strengths to achieve goals together. It's basically the "two heads are better than one" philosophy, which so often proves true. In simulated work exercises, teams experience the benefits of working together.

Likewise, the faith community staff forms a ministry team by combining their various skills and abilities to work together toward a common faith vision or mission. You will be part of that team. As you plan your work, keep this overall ministry vision in mind. All that you do should contribute toward this larger goal of helping people deepen their faith and live it out in their daily lives. Utilize your team members' expertise as well as willingly offering your skills and knowledge to the team.

SUMMARY

Remember that developing a health ministry is a team effort, one that involves the whole faith community. Your role as a leader is to inspire, motivate, and enable others to help you in your work. Establish a health committee to help you plan, prioritize, and carry out your ministry. This group will also help you market and interpret the ministry to the congregation. They will be your cheerleaders and advocates. They will have invested in your work and your position and will support you and celebrate with you.

Working with volunteers is one of the great joys of faith community nursing. You will get to know many people this way and make some very good friends. It is rewarding to help others find their niche in ministry and develop in other ways, including spiritually. Together you'll help many people toward the goal of better health. If you pay attention to the best ways to recruit, retain, and reward volunteers, you will truly feel as though health ministry is a team effort and you will be seen as a good leader, all of which will have a positive impact on your practice.

REFERENCES AND RESOURCES

All online references and resources were current September 30, 2008.

REFERENCES

American Nurses Association (ANA) and Health Ministries Association (HMA). 2005. *Faith community nursing: Scope and standards of practice.* Silver Spring, MD: Nursesbooks.org.

SUGGESTED RESOURCES

Health Ministries Association. 2002. *A guide to developing a health ministry.* Roswell, GA: Health Ministries Association.

Huber, D. 2000. *Leadership and nursing care management,* 2nd ed. Philadelphia: W.B. Saunders.

Kouzes, J., and B. Posner. 2003. *The leadership challenge,* 3rd ed. New York: Jossey-Bass.

Marquis, B., C. Huston, M. Cantu, and C. Huston. 2002. *Leadership roles and management functions in nursing: Theory and application,* 4th ed. Baltimore, MD: Lippincott Williams and Wilkins.

Sullivan, E., and P. Decker. 2005. *Effective leadership and management in nursing.* Upper Saddle River, NJ: Pearson Prentice Hall.

Yoder-Wise, P. 2001. *Leading and managing in nursing,* 3rd ed. St. Louis, MO: Mosby.

ORGANIZATIONAL RESOURCES

The BeFriender Program (Pastoral care lay training): **www.befrienderministry.org**

Stephen Ministries Program (Lay ministry training): **www.stephenministries.org**

CHAPTER 7

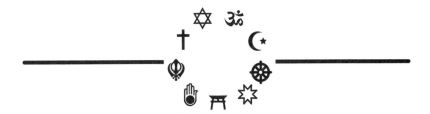

THE HEALTHY TREE:
KEEPING YOURSELF HEALTHY

SINCE ONE OF THE THINGS THIS CHAPTER is about is making time to play, I'd like you to draw a picture. Find yourself a big sheet of paper and some crayons or felt-tip markers. No, you don't have to be an artist. First, think of your favorite kind of tree. Where is the tree located? What is its shape and appearance? Do you picture it during a particular season? Are any animals or people associated with the tree? Now sketch a picture of what you consider to be a healthy tree. Take your time and just enjoy putting down on paper the visual images that come to mind.

When you're done, talk about your drawing with someone. Tell the person about your tree and identify and describe its healthy characteristics. Then, using these descriptions, write down a definition of wholistic health.

What insights about health do you get from doing this simple and fun activity?

Reflect a bit on the following questions. Is your tree perfect or does it have some broken branches? Perhaps there is a burl on the trunk or one of the branches. This is a knotty growth that is a response to an earlier injury. It is prized by wood turners for its interesting grain patterns. What impact do broken branches and unusual growths have on trees? What are the implications of brokenness and illness on human health?

Did you draw roots for your tree? Are they shallow or deep? How do these characteristics apply to a person's health, especially to their spiritual foundations? Write down your thoughts about these and other ideas that come to mind in comparing and contrasting a healthy tree with your own health.

I learned this exercise from a psychiatric–mental health nurse at a district nursing meeting years ago, and because I thought it was particularly meaningful for faith community nursing, I had our program's new FCNs do it as part of the class on wholistic health. They subsequently used it in faith community presentations as an excellent and enjoyable way to get people thinking and talking about the many dimensions and meanings of whole-person health.

The following are some of the ideas this exercise generates for me. Just as your tree requires food and water, you, too, must take care of your physical needs—eating properly, getting exercise and adequate rest. Like a tree that bends in the wind, you must be flexible, adapting to changing situations. Just as nutrients are conveyed from the tree roots to its branches, feeding your spiritual roots with love, beauty, spiritual study, prayer, and meditation will nourish all of the body. The analogies from a tree's health to your own health are many, but I think you get the idea. Remember these elements of a healthy tree as you take care of your own health.

BALANCE AND BOUNDARIES

I don't know if my first few months as an FCN are typical, but I do know that my perfectionist nature is not uncommon among nurses. In addition to working 20 hours a week in the faith community, I spent time at home reading and planning for future programs. Even over a two-week family vacation, I prepared for the weight management support group I would start upon my return. When I began to feel overworked and underpaid, I realized I needed a better balance in my life. I made some decisions about work that were important to taking care of my own physical and mental health. Although I still thought about work as creative ideas popped into my mind at all hours of the day, I took less of the job home and vowed never to spend another vacation absorbed with work. This new balance was refreshing and resulted in a better attitude toward my work.

Another way to keep some boundaries on your work is to let the faith community know that you do not regularly take calls at home. Encourage people to call you at work or to make an appointment to see you during your office hours. One FCN I know wears her lab coat if she is working; when she is not wearing her lab coat, e.g., during the main worship day, this communicates that she is there just as a member—so if people have issues they need to discuss, they can use the phone message line. This helps delineate, for the faith community, the FCN's boundaries between her "working self" and her "personal self."

New FCNs may feel, as I did, that they have to continually develop new programs that will show health ministry's worth. To some extent, this is necessary because health ministry is inherently invisible, taking place in people's homes, on the phone, or in the office. And it is true that people often question what faith community staff do all day. So there is that pressure to make faith community nursing visible, especially the first year, through classes, support groups, and health fairs. Since a certain amount of visibility is necessary, think of some activities you can do regularly that don't take much preparation, such as blood pressure screening, so that the congregation sees you at work.

But before you get caught up in working well beyond your allotted hours, take time to plan a balanced life for yourself. One way to assess and visualize how you are spending your time is to draw what is called a Pie of Life. Draw a circle for a 24-hour day and divide it, like a pie, into sections that are proportionate to the time you spend in each daily activity, such as work, sleep, and play. When you're done, compare the sizes of each section. You may be surprised that your play slice is so small. If the portions are not the size you would like, think of ways to resize them to achieve a better balance.

ACCEPT HELP AND SEEK SUPPORT

It is easy for nurses to want to do more and more. Nurses are naturally caring people, and people's needs are unending. Since FCNs are responsible for the hours they keep, it makes it even easier to keep working. Sometimes the problem is that we think we are the only ones who can do the work, and we forget that others can help us. Especially in health ministry, we need to be intentional about involving the faith community in our work. As we discussed in the last chapter, nurture that group of volunteers interested in your work and willing to help you. Realize that you need to use the spiritual gifts and talents of others to achieve the best health ministry results.

Also, be aware of and access your support networks. If your position is supported by a healthcare institution, you may have a faith community nursing program supervisor available to help you with work concerns, advocate for you, and advise you. The faith community's senior spiritual leadership staff, especially your supervisor, should be one of your main supporters. If you need to meet with them at a time other than your weekly meeting, make an appointment. This respects their busy schedules. Develop your relationships with the members of your health committee and let them know how much their support and encouragement mean to you. The health committee can be a group that looks out for your health and well-being and upholds you and the health ministry in prayer. Find other FCNs in your area with whom you can meet and talk. If you are the only FCN in town, contact the IPNRC or HMA to locate other FCNs you can reach by phone or e-mail.

FCN Carol Hamilton, who has ongoing support through a hospital program, says this about the monthly meetings with the other FCNs in her area:

> Not only can we share common concerns but also resource information in our community and just plain encouragement and understanding of the challenges. I would certainly suggest to anyone beginning faith community nursing that they find a network of support with other FCNs, if at all possible, and if not, at least an accountability group of folks that really understand the faith/health connection and what faith community nursing is all about.

Principles for Keeping Yourself Healthy

- Maintain good health habits.
- Nourish your spiritual roots daily.
- Know and maintain your caregiving limits and boundaries.
- Take time to play, laugh, and relax each day.
- Develop and use your support systems.
- Involve others in health ministry.

SPIRITUAL NURTURE

Just as a tree's roots must have enough water and minerals to sustain its growth and development, nourishing your spiritual roots contributes to wholistic health. Scientific evidence is accumulating on the ways a belief system impacts health (Ray 2004). Since our spiritual belief system is connected to our endocrine, nervous, and immune systems, we strengthen our overall health when we strengthen our belief system. We do this through positive attitudes, values, relationships, and emotions as well as by taking time each day to grow in our faith. How will you feed your spiritual roots? Are you making space for spirituality in your life? If you don't plan for daily prayer or meditation and spiritual study, it's easy to get to the end of the day and find you've run out of both time and energy to do those important things. Keep your spiritual plan realistic, but block out one or two times during the day when you can be by yourself and in a quiet place for prayer and study. Perhaps you have time in the morning for reading some scripture or religious material and silence for listening to your inner source of wisdom. At the end of the day you might want to do some journaling or listening to sacred music. Whatever ways you choose, spending time meditating and reflecting is essential to good health.

What else refreshes your spirit? My husband and I just returned from our faith community's retreat in the beautiful green mountains of western North Carolina. We worshiped together, talked with our friends while rocking on the cabins' front porches, hiked up the old logging road to enjoy the gorgeous view of the sparkling lake, and viewed the beautiful quilts displayed on the buildings' walls. I consider all these activities spiritual. The German writer, Goethe, gives similar advice: "[E]very day....hear a little song, read a good poem, see a fine picture...." Think of all the everyday ways you can nourish your spirit.

Ways to Nurture Your Spirit

- Regularly practice spiritual disciplines, such as prayer and worship, which are important to your particular faith.
- Read and study religious materials.
- Attend religious workshops and conferences.
- Go on a spiritual retreat.
- Enroll in a spiritual formation program.
- Work with a spiritual director.
- Enjoy the arts: music, dance, theater, painting, and other creative arts. Develop your own creativity.
- Enjoy nature and the out-of-doors: watch the birds, take a walk, plant a garden.
- Develop loving and healthy relationships with others.
- Care for a pet animal.

Consider some extra spiritual nourishment every few years by asking your faith community to allow you to go on sabbatical. It's not unusual for spiritual leaders to take a sabbatical leave of a few months after several years of work. For an FCN, the leave may only be a week and may not be a paid leave. Even if not fully paid, the faith community might cover the sabbatical expenses, such as conference or study tuition. Carol Tippe, an FCN in Iowa, was able to take a four-month sabbatical after working 10 years. The faith community paid for expenses associated with this time of spiritual growth, study, and Sabbath rest. Carol says, "I am the first parish FCN to have a sabbatical! I am ready for another!!! It was a great experience!! It included spiritual direction time too." To read more about Carol's sabbatical, go to her web site: www.nursing.uiowa.edu/sites/users/Ctippe/sabbat.htm.

Using all these means to grow spiritually not only refreshes you and helps you to stay healthy, but they will also give you greater confidence in fulfilling the spiritual role of faith community nursing.

FINDING A RHYTHM

Don't be concerned if your beginning work schedule feels rather inefficient. Faith community nursing does not have the regular hours you may be used to in a previous nursing position. It will take a few weeks before you realize a certain pattern to your work week. Unlike most nursing schedules, determining your schedule as an FCN is largely your responsibility. Eventually your activities will be more predictable and you'll be able to plan your week better. Just try to arrange your hours as efficiently as possible.

It's especially important for FCNs working part-time to group activities together as much as possible. Otherwise, part-time hours can quickly become full-time. Be aware of which meetings (staff, pastoral care, and committee) you need to attend, and schedule other activities on those days rather than making a special trip just for a meeting.

What you plan and when you schedule it will depend on many factors. For instance, I found that most people, especially those in the hospital or nursing homes, like visits either in the late morning or early afternoon. Educational programs need to be planned around work schedules and night-driving limitations. For working people, programs are usually held in the evening, while older persons, many of whom no longer drive at night because of vision problems, prefer to attend during the day.

Working on the day the faith community worships together will be a new experience for most of you. As a faith community member you may have taught religious education classes or had other responsibilities in addition to worship on that day, but as an FCN you'll be at work even during the worship service, responding to the occasional medical emergency or talking to people before and after the service. People will ask you health questions or want to share concerns with you either about themselves or others. Therefore, since this day becomes a work day, be sure to include these hours in your weekly total.

If you're working in your own faith community, you may not want to be on duty as the FCN during the main worship day. If this is the case, be sure to inform the faith community. As noted earlier, one FCN wears her lab coat to indicate when she is working; when she is not wearing her lab coat, this communicates that she is there just as a member.

A FEW FINAL SUGGESTIONS FOR KEEPING YOURSELF HEALTHY

Remember that you are not expected to heal the world! You only have to be faithful to your particular ministry. It also helps to learn to distinguish between being responsible *to* others, rather than *for* others. There *is* a difference! You are responsible to foster whole-person health through teaching, health counseling, and connecting people to resources, but each person is responsible for making his or her own choices in life. In all you do, keep in mind that you want to keep people from becoming dependent on you. Allow them to take responsibility for their health and their life choices as partners with you in all aspects of their health care.

If you are always thinking about work, feeling overburdened or unduly fatigued, you may be assuming too much responsibility for people's actions, behaviors, and choices. Step back a moment and evaluate how you are getting your needs for love and a sense of accomplishment met. Is it through friends, family, hobby, volunteer or community activity, or is it only through the people you care for? Recognize how to meet your own needs so that you are not meeting them only through your ministry.

You may fear failing at ministry. However, the only way you can *fail* at ministry is not to learn from your experiences. Michelle Pearce, FCN, puts it this way: "I have found that it is my honest and sincere desire to assist people and serve and also the power of presence that are the most valuable assets I bring to the church and the people."

TAKING TIME TO REFLECT

Taking time to reflect on your ministry by using a spiritual or theological reflection method can help you care for yourself and others. It will provide insights into your own behavior and help you respond to people's needs in the most healthy and helpful way. One theological reflection method I used with our FCNs was developed by Peter Buttitta (1992) especially for FCNs. It works this way: one FCN comes to the group prepared to talk about a recent personal or professional concern. These are the next five steps:

1. The FCN describes the basic facts of the situation.

2. The FCN relates feelings associated with the experience.

3. The FCN forms a metaphor from these facts and feelings. For instance, the experience may make one feel like being "drowned in a storm-tossed sea."

4. The spiritual leader guides group discussion of this image to arrive at spiritual insight. This insight helps clarify and challenge the FCN's questions, attitudes, beliefs, perceptions, and ways of acting. It also suggests particular actions to be taken.

5. The FCN applies this insight to the present situation or to a similar one in the future.

At the heart of this method is discovering and responding to spiritual guidance in daily experience.

HEALING AND HEALING SERVICES

Healing and helping people to become whole are at the heart of faith community nursing. Nursing, in general, is closely connected in people's minds with healing. In recent years, many faith communities have once again made healing an integral part of their work and worship. One example is the American Jewish healing movement that began within the past two decades. The movement has taken several forms (Sered 2005). A variety of private practices and group settings engage with illness and healing from a Jewish perspective. Some of these practices and settings are highly traditional, such as personal prayer in the context of the standard daily or Sabbath liturgy, and during the customary lighting of Sabbath candles. Other practices include:

• Integration of Jewish sacred objects, healing songs, prayers, and symbols into eclectic healing repertoires that for an individual may include guided visualizations, meditation, or other personally significant elements

- Prayer for the Sick ceremonies during the Sabbath morning service
- Synagogue-sponsored healing services
- Independent healing practitioners
- Twelve Step groups (such as AA)
- Hospital chaplaincy

This list will look familiar to many Christian faith groups. My own Episcopal congregation offers prayers for the sick during the Sunday worship service and healing prayers after the service for individuals with laying-on of hands and anointing with oil. We also have two healing services a week, one during the day and one in the evening. During the evening healing service our healing team provides individual *soaking prayer*. The term *soaking prayer* was initiated by our priest to emphasize the need and benefit of ongoing prayer for healing.

People will particularly see the FCN as a symbol of health and healing. In that regard, if the faith community you're working in has a healing service, it is natural for you to be involved in it. You may want to counsel people about their health concerns in private before or after the service. If it is appropriate or allowed by the faith community, you may participate in the service itself as a part of the healing team. There may be special training available for you to do this, such as the Christian resource, The International Order of St. Luke.

If your faith community does not have a healing service, you can talk with the senior spiritual leadership staff about starting one. Some senior spiritual leaders are reluctant to have healing services because of their sometimes sensationalist history and people's expectations of instant physical healing. These fears can be addressed by educating the faith community about healing. Just as illness often develops over time, it also takes time for healing to occur. Healing is not only physical. Memories and relationships are healed as well. Jackie Herzlinger, FCN, writes this about healing: "I don't pray for cure; I pray for healing—emotional wholeness, help with difficult situations." A faith community's healing ministry is a natural complement to its health ministry. Find out your faith community's attitude on healing and what resources are available to help start this important ministry.

Participating in a healing ministry may make you aware of your own need for healing. Hurts that are not healed may keep you from being effective in your ministry. One nurse I interviewed for an FCN position told me at length about the physical abuse she endured from her former husband. It was evident that her emotional wounds were not healed sufficiently for her to minister to others in a similar situation. However, once our wounds are healed, they can make us better healers. This is Henri Nouwen's message of the *wounded healer* (Nouwen 1979). As we experience healing of physical illness or inner hurts, we are better able to understand others' struggles and help them in the healing process.

SUMMARY

Because the most important tool in your ministry is yourself, it is important to take good care of that tool. Sometimes when you feel inadequate for the ministry task, you may think you need more and more tools, such as more knowledge, or that you just need to work harder and harder. Try to recognize when you are falling into this trap. Remember to call on your spiritual source of power to work with and through you. Don't forget that faith community nursing is more about *being* than *doing*.

Like most ministry, faith community nursing happens one person at a time. It is a quiet and often invisible ministry. Unless someone receives help from you, or hears about it from a friend, many people will not know about your work. Of course, you'll work to communicate what you do, but the value of what you do is not based on how much you do. Take pleasure in the relationships you build, the things you learn, and the way you grow and develop spiritually. Celebrate the small steps people take toward better physical, mental, and spiritual health, and the ways they learn to care for each other. Take care of yourself. Most of all, enjoy the journey of faith community nursing.

REFERENCES AND RESOURCES

All online references and resources were current September 30, 2008.

REFERENCES

Buttitta, P. 1992. *The still, small voice that beckons: A theological reflection method for health ministry.* Chicago: Reflection Resources.

Nouwen, H. 1979. *The wounded healer.* New York: Image Books.

Ray, O. 2004. How the mind hurts and heals the body. *American Psychologist* 59 (1):1–12.

Sered, S. 2005. Bodies and souls: Jewish healing in America. *Pastoral Sciences* 24 (2): 81–95.

SUGGESTED RESOURCES

Benson, H., and E. Stuart. 1992. *The wellness book.* New York: Simon and Schuster.

Boss, J. 1994. Caring for ourselves: Being a professional caretaker can be dangerous to your health. *Health and Development*: Issue 4:10–14.

Burkhardt, M., and M. Nagai-Jacobsen. 2002. *Spirituality—Living our connectedness.* Albany, NY: Delmar.

Canham, E. 1999. *Heart whispers: Benedictine wisdom for today.* Nashville: Upper Room.

Craig, C. 2004. Spiritual health. In R. Daniels, ed. *Nursing fundamentals: Caring and critical decision making*, pp. 1489–1508. Clifton Park, New York: Delmar.

Dossey, B., and L. Keegan. 2000. Self-assessments: Facilitating healing in self and others. In B. Dossey, et al., *Holistic nursing: A handbook for practice*, 3rd ed., pp. 361–74. Gaithersburg, MD: Aspen.

Dossey, L. 1993. *Healing words.* San Francisco: Harper.

Foster, R. 1998. *Celebration of discipline.* San Francisco: Harper

_____. 1992. *Prayer: Finding the heart's true home.* San Francisco: Harper.

Foster, R., and J. Smith, eds. 1993. *Devotional classics.* San Francisco: Harper.

Groer, M. 2001. Spirituality and holistic nursing. In D. Wilt and C. Smucker, eds., *Nursing the spirit,* pp. 19–29. Washington, DC: American Nurses Publishing.

Hankinson, S., G. Coldita, J. Manson, and F. Speizer, eds. 2001. *Healthy women, healthy lives.* New York: Simon and Schuster.

Henry, L., and J. Henry. 2004. *The soul of the caring nurse.* Washington, DC: American Nurses Publishing.

James, D., and E. Whitehead. 1995. *Method in ministry: Theological reflection and Christian ministry.* New York: Seabury.

Kabat-Zinn, J. 1994. *Wherever you go there you are: Mindfulness meditation in everyday life.* New York: Hyperion.

Keegan, L. 1994. *The nurse as healer.* Albany, NY: Delmar.

Kidd, S. 1990. *When the heart waits: Spiritual direction for life's sacred questions.* San Francisco: Harper.

Kinast, R. 1991. *Let the ministry teach: A handbook for theological reflection.* Madeira Beach, FL: Center for Theological Reflection.

Lauterbach, S., and P. Becker. 1998. Caring for self: Becoming a self-reflective nurse. In C. Guzzetta, ed., *Essential readings in holistic nursing,* pp. 97–107. Gaithersburg, MD: Aspen.

MacNutt, F. 2001. *The power to heal.* Notre Dame, IN: Ave Maria Press.

McKivergin, M. 2000. The nurse as an instrument of healing. In B. Dossey, et al., eds., *Holistic nursing: A handbook for practice,* 3rd ed., pp. 207–227. Gaithersburg, MD: Aspen.

Moyers, B. 1990. *Healing and the mind.* New York: Doubleday.

Nouwen, H. 1997. *Spiritual journals.* New York: Continuum.

Patterson, D. 2003. *The essential parish nurse: ABCs for congregational health ministry.* New York: The Pilgrim Press.

_____. 2005. *Healing words for healing people: Prayers and meditations for parish nurses and other health professionals.* Berea, OH: Pilgrim.

Pearson, M. 2000. *Christian healing: A practical and comprehensive guide.* Grand Rapids, MI: Chosen Books.

Pennington, M. 1998. *Lectio divina: Renewing the ancient practice of praying the scriptures.* New York: Crossroad.

Postema, D. 1997. *Catch your breath: God's invitation to Sabbath rest.* Grand Rapids, MI: Faith Alive.

_____. 1983. *Space for God: The study and practice of prayer and spirituality.* Grand Rapids, MI: Bible Way.

Remen, N. 1996. In the service of life. *Noetic Sciences Review.* Issue 37 (Spring): 24–25.

_____. 1996. *Kitchen table wisdom: Stories that heal.* New York: Riverhead.

Rupp, J. 1992. *May I have this dance?* Notre Dame, IN: Ave Maria Press.

Sanford, A. 1972. *The healing light.* New York: Ballantine.

Wilkinson, J. 1998. *The Bible and healing.* Grand Rapids, MI: Wm. B. Eerdmans.

ORGANIZATIONAL RESOURCES

The International Order of St. Luke the Physician is an interdenominational Christian fellowship dedicated to the healing ministry of Jesus Christ: **www.orderofstluke.org**

CHAPTER 8

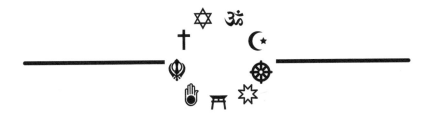

A MODEL OF JEWISH CONGREGATIONAL NURSING

LINDA WEINBERG, PhD, RN, NP, ET

ORIGINS OF JEWISH CONGREGATIONAL MODEL

Not long after I took a course on parish nursing at Villanova University in Villanova, Pennsylvania, in 1997, I realized the model created by Rev. Granger Westberg could not be applied entirely to the philosophy and theology of the various Jewish communities in the United States.

Inspired by the course, I established a parish nursing practice in my synagogue in Phoenixville, Pennsylvania. Almost immediately, my fellow congregants asked questions about the title of the program: parish nursing. Parish nursing does not exist as a term or concept in the Jewish religion.

My rabbi and I thought it more appropriate to change the term from parish nursing to Jewish congregational nursing (JCN). This new name made more sense to my fellow congregants, and they began to participate in programs created under the JCN umbrella. The Hebrew word for JCN is Ha-yehoodeet (Ha-keheelah Akh ot).

Whether it was called parish nursing or Jewish Congregational Nursing, I still performed the seven key functions of a faith-based community nurse:

1. Health educator
2. Integrator of faith and health
3. Referral agent
4. Personal health counselor
5. Coordinator of volunteers
6. Health advocate
7. Developer of support groups

These seven functions were always carried out with a "Jewish twist." I worked with the rabbi (rav), the health board (va'ad bree' ot), and the surrounding Jewish and non-Jewish community (keheelah) to create an effective and successful Jewish congregational practice in my geographical area.

As the years went by, I was anxious to educate other Jewish nurses about JCN in the surrounding states of New York, New Jersey, and Delaware. At the time, no funding was available to offer such as course. With the rabbi's blessing and cooperation, I began to think about offering a course at my synagogue. My colleagues at Villanova University allowed me to use their course materials on parish nursing. As a result, each participant in the JCN course would receive 35 CEU credits. At this point, I breathed a sigh of relief that the bulk of the work needed to organize the course for Jewish nurses was mostly done. Soon after, however, I realized that I could not teach a JCN course based solely on the content taken from a parish nursing course at a Catholic university.

The focus on health and healing in the parish nursing model conceived by Rev. Granger Westberg is rooted in the Judeo-Christian Old Testament, which does not separate the spiritual from the physical aspects of healing. But it is also modeled on Jesus's ministry of healing and preaching described in the New Testament.

Although the teaching of Jesus is respected by people of all religions, it does not figure in Jewish theology or tradition. I concluded that it was necessary to develop a Model of Jewish Congregational Nursing (MJCN) based on the thousands of years of Jewish history, theology, philosophy, and traditions. This Model of Jewish congregational nursing could then be used with the American Nurses Association and Health Ministries Association's *Faith Community Nursing: Scope and Standards of Practice* (ANA and HMA 2005) when providing this type of nursing care.

The first course in Jewish congregational nursing was held at Congregational B'Nai Jacob in Phoenixville, Pennsylvania, on March 3, 10, 17, and 24, and April 7, 2002. The twelve participating nurses came from New York, New Jersey, and Pennsylvania and represented Reform, Conservative, Orthodox, and Reconstruction denominations.

CONFIGURATION OF THE MODEL OF JEWISH CONGREGATIONAL NURSING

The six-pointed Model of Jewish congregational nursing is contained within a larger circle that represents the socio-economic, political, cultural, and spiritual communities in which Jewish congregational nursing can occur. The Star of David (Magen David) was chosen to represent this model graphically because it is the universally recognized symbol of Judaism.

The first known mention in the literature of the six-pointed star was in 300 C.E. on a tombstone in Southern Italy. Later King Carl VI ordered the Jews living in Prague to make a flag for themselves that contained a six-pointed star (Magen David) and the five-pointed star of King Solomon. The Magen David was carried on the six-sided shields that King David's soldiers carried into battle. According to the Kabbalah, the book of Jewish mysticism, the number six represents the six directions: east, west, north, south, heavens, and earth. Six letters are also contained in the Hebrew word for Magen David. In addition, the 12 sides of the Magen David represent the 12 tribes of Israel.

A later scholar, Franz Rosensweig, suggested that the top part of the triangle represents a striving toward God and Heaven and the lower triangle represents the treading downward toward the real world (Bleck 1999, p. 349). The metaphor of striving in opposing directions is an important one for the Jewish congregational nurse. The nurse is striving to give the highest level of nursing care while the patient is living daily with life's physical and spiritual struggles.

The mission of the Jewish congregational nurse is to infuse Jewish history, philosophy, theology, and traditions, as well as ideas about health and illness, into the seven functions of the congregational nurse. This infusion serves two purposes: The first purpose is to allow the recipient of JCN care to "maintain physical health and vigor that his soul may be upright in order to serve God" (Maimonides, Mishnah Torah, Doet. 3.3). The second purpose is to establish the Model of Jewish Congregational Nursing as a distinct and unique part of faith community nursing.

EXPLANATION OF THE MODEL OF JEWISH CONGREGATIONAL NURSING

The following is an explanation of the individual components in the six-pointed Magen David. (See its illustration on the next page.) The explanation proceeds from the top of the model clockwise, starting at the north (tsafon), going east (meezrakhah), then south (darom), and finally to the west (ma'arv). This method of explanation reflects four of the six points expressed in Kabbalistic thought. The two remaining points which include the rabbi (rav), the health board (va'ad bree'ot), and the community (keeheelah), will be explained after the concept of communal responsibility (arvot) has been discussed below.

1. LISTEN (SHEMA)

Shema, the Hebrew word for *hear*, is located at the northern part of the MJCN. Placing the word, Shema, at the top of the model was done deliberately for three reasons.

The first reason is that listening, or being present, is an essential key to effective nursing everywhere. In reality, nursing care may be done without paying 100 percent attention to that particular individual. But caring about that person, which results in more effective physical and spiritual attentiveness, can only be accomplished if the nurse "pays heed" or "lends an ear" to a significant message that requires attention (Lamm 1998, p. 13).

The second reason is because the Shema is the name of the most significant prayer relating to Jewish identification—be it an individual or entire community. It represents the ideals of hope, courage, and commitment (Lamm 1998, p. 4). The Shema begins as follows: "Hear O Israel: the Lord is our God, the Lord is one...."

The following story is told by the Holocaust historian, Yaffa Eliach (Yaffa Eliach Collection, Center for Holocaust Studies, Museum of Jewish Heritage, New York, New York). After World War II, an American Jew went to Europe to look for Jewish children. To find the Jewish children in the various institutions that he visited, the American Jew began to recite the Shema. If the children were Jewish, they began to come out and walk toward the man who was trying to find them.

The third reason that Shema is placed at the most northern part of the MJCN is that it exemplifies one of the more important debates in Judaism: the debate between Jewish law (Halaka) and Jewish spirituality (Ruhanee). Jewish law originated in the oral law and became written law as contained in the Gemara and Mishnah. This written law later became the Talmud. The Talmud was then codified by later rabbis (Lamm 1998, p. 6).

Spirituality ranges from daily reflections about who we are to more abstract notions found in such works as the Kabbalah, the book of Jewish mysticism. While spirituality is subjective, individualistic, and "in the moment," law is objective and requires order and obedience (Lamm 1998, p. 6).

Judaism values both spirituality and law simultaneously. Rather than allow one to override the other, a Jew is expected to respect both. A balance (ma'azlan) in one's life is of paramount concern to both the Jew and Jewish congregational nurse.

CASE STUDY: BALANCE IN JEWISH CONGREGATIONAL NURSING (MA'AZLAN)

A Jewish congregational nurse is on her way to synagogue for Yom Kippur services. Yom Kippur, Day of Atonement, is one of the most important holidays of the Jewish calendar year. As required by Jewish Law, it is set aside for praying, attending services, fasting, and refraining from everyday activities, including work.

The nurse gets a call from the daughter of one of the synagogue's congregants. Her mother has just fallen and she is requesting that the nurse make a home visit immediately. The Jewish congregational nurse knows what the law and observances mean to her and the congregants of the synagogue. But she is expected, in her role as Jewish congregational nurse, to merge the law and the vision of spirituality into a daily practice that benefits the recipient of this particular type of nursing care. Therefore, she tells the patient's daughter that she will make a home visit as soon as possible—Yom Kippur or not—for the nurse has "heard" what the congregant's daughter has said and has acted according to her own spirituality.

2. PRAYER OF HEALING (MI SHE-BERAKH)

Jewish ideas about health can be found in Biblical sources and subsequently in both textual and folk interpretations of these sources (Praglin 1999). Ancient Jews believed God to be the only one who could heal them. In fact, God was viewed as the source of health and illness (Praglin 1999). Illness was seen as either an individual or communal punishment, rather than a demonic

JEWISH CONGREGATIONAL NURSING

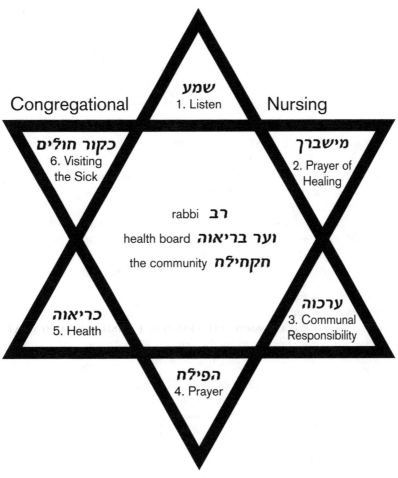

Congregational   Nursing

שמע
1. Listen

כקור חולים
6. Visiting
the Sick

מישברך
2. Prayer of
Healing

rabbi רב
health board ועד בריאוה
the community חקחילה

כריאוה
5. Health

ערכוה
3. Communal
Responsibility

הפילח
4. Prayer

1. Shema שמע (Listen)	Core prayer of Judaism
2. Mi she-Berakh מישברך (Prayer of Healing)	Fusion of mind and body through prayer, art, communication from person to person.
3. Arvot ערכוה (Communal Responsibility)	Pirkei Avot. All of Israel are responsible for one another.
4. Tefelah הפילח (Prayer)	Consists of historical texts and prayers. Concerned with communication with G-d.
5. Bree'oot כריאוה (Health)	"Maintain physical health and vigor that his soul may be upright in order to serve G-d." (Maimonides, Mishnah Torah, Deuteronomy 3:3)
6. Bikur Cholim כקור חולים (Visiting the Sick)	G-d through his messengers visiting Abraham after his circumcision. (Genesis 12:13)

© Linda Weinberg 2008

force (Kee 1992, p. 659). Similarly, healing was associated with individual or communal restoration, forgiveness, renewal, reward, or deliverance from destruction (Kee 1992, p. 659).

The Bible has many references to both physical and spiritual healing that the ancient Jews believed led to wholeness. In Genesis 20:17, God healed Abimelech after Abraham pleaded for his recovery. If Israel kept the Ten Commandments, God promised to keep the people of Israel healthy (Exodus 15:26). Moses pleaded for his sister Miriam's life in Deuteronomy 32:39. God said, "I deal death and give life. I wounded and I will heal. None can deliver my hand." Other ideas and statements about healing can be found throughout Jewish texts.

In the post-Biblical period, Jewish ideas of health and healing were found in the Talmud (law), the Mishnah (written views of the rabbis), and the Midrash (legends). The Talmud contained a prohibition that Jews could not live in a place that did not have physician services. The rabbis interpreted Exodus (21:19–20) saying that God himself authorized—in fact, required—medicine and healing, "so that the victim of injury could be thoroughly healed" (Praglin 1999, p. 3). Sections of the Mishnah mandate that every Jew is both legally and practically bound to maintain his or her body with proper diet, exercise, hygiene, sleep, and sexual relations. In the Midrash, B. Yoma 82, mental health was to be treated as seriously as physical health. In fact, a threat to mental health (teruf da'af) was deemed to be treated the same as a threat to one's physical life (piku'ah nefesh) (Feldman 1986, p. 8).

These three texts—the Talmud, Mishnah, and Midrash—maintained that God was the sole healer. Physicians, nurses, visitors, and hospitals were regarded as partners and agents of God, but not as substitutes. Since God was viewed as the sole healer or the ultimate physician, petitionary prayers to heal the sick were offered to God three times a day during the morning, afternoon, and evening traditional services.

The Mi she-Berakh prayer is representative of the importance of the role that health plays in the everyday lives of Jews. Therefore, it was chosen as an essential part of the MJCN. The prayer begins as follows: "O God, who blessed our ancestors, Abraham, Issac, and Jacob, Sarah, Rebekah, Rachel, and Leah, send your blessings to _____ ...."

3A. COMMUNAL RESPONSIBILITY (ARVOT) – OUTER ASPECT

The theme of community responsibility is one of the cornerstones of the Jewish religion. From ancient times until the present, whether contained in the written or oral law, the theme is found not only in texts but also within the mission of Jewish organizations throughout the world.

The first-century scholar, Rabbi Hillel, a man known for his kindness and patience, was asked by a non-Jew to be taught the entire Torah "on one foot." Hillel regarded this request as a monumental one and chose not to turn the man away. Rabbi Hillel told the man that the most important idea in Judaism is that you treat your fellow man as you would like to be treated.

The non-Jew in this well-known story knew that Judaism required service to both human beings and God. But he is asking Rabbi Hillel which is more important: service to God or service to human beings. Is Judaism God- or human-centered? Rabbi Hillel responded to this man, "If I am forced to make a choice, let me tell you God is more interested in people being good to each other than in worshipping Him. God can always manage..." (Bleck 1999, pp. 37–38).

3B. COMMUNAL RESPONSIBILITY (ARVOT) – INNER ASPECT

So pivotal a concept is communal responsibility to the MJCN that it is placed on one of the outer points of the Magen David, as well as in the innermost portion of the Magen David itself. As it pertains to the MJCN, the community consists of the rabbi (rav), health board (va'ad bree'oot), and the community (keheelah), defined as both Jewish and non-Jewish.

Judaism is not a hierarchical religion. Very little distinction is made between the lay leadership and the rabbinate. An ordinary Jew can lead a funeral worship service. Actually, the only thing that a rabbi can do in front of a congregation that cannot be done by a layperson is to sign a marriage license. And that power is not granted by Jewish law, but by the secular state in which the rabbi lives. The rabbi is regarded as a teacher, informed in areas of traditional liturgy, cultural principles, and law.

As a result, the MJCN can function with or without a rabbi, with or without a synagogue, in a community center, or anywhere in the community. Many areas in this country and throughout the world do not have even a part-time rabbi. Some congregations have no permanent home in which to meet and instead rotate from one congregant's home to another. The idea that an MJCN can function only with a rabbi does not reflect the traditions or reality of contemporary Jews throughout the world.

What is essential to the functioning of the MJCN is a committed and caring group of Jewish people who appreciate the intertwining of Judaism's long-standing textual traditions and philosophies regarding health and their impact upon a person's soul and faith. Such a group would organize themselves into a health board or va'ad bree'ot. The number of people who might serve on this health board is not a fixed number. As we all know, four hard-working, committed, and interested people in any situation can accomplish far more than twenty not-so-hard-working, not-so-committed, and not-so-interested people.

It is also essential that the people who serve on this health board (va'ad bree'ot) must be able to listen (leha'azeen) and hear (shemm'ee) each other, the members of the community, and the Jewish congregational nurse.

The relationship among the rabbi, health board, community, and JCN in the MJCN is a circular one. It might be that the rabbi starts an initiative and the rest follow. Or it may be that the JCN begins a dialogue between the rabbi, health board, and community, which again reflects the non-hierarchical nature of Judaism.

CASE STUDY: COMMUNITY LISTENING AND RESPONSIBILITY IN MJCN

So many possibilities came to mind when I first established myself as the Jewish congregational nurse for my medium-sized synagogue. As Robert Frost once said, there are two paths in the woods. Which one to pick?

With my rabbi's support, I began to seek out various members of my congregation who might be interested in working with me to establish various health programs that would merge Jewish views on health with Jewish views on spirituality. I found four people, professionals and nonprofessionals, who were committed in both their ideas and time.

With my background in public health, I began to look at my synagogue, the institution, as my client and not at the individual congregants. As with any other client, my synagogue had members of all ages. These members had several things in common—for example, a lack of exercise and excess weight. I met with the rabbi and the health board and proposed two programs for both the congregation and the outlying communities. Both programs integrated health and spirituality, although "spirituality" was not defined in these programs as only Jewish in nature. Weekly classes in both yoga and Tai Chi began, with the approval of both the rabbi and health board. Both Jews and non-Jews participated in these programs which were open to the larger community. Eight people signed up for the eight-week course in yoga and 10 people signed up for the eight-week course in Tai Chi. The fees were more reasonable than those at the surrounding gyms. Attendance was 90 percent throughout the sessions. After each exercise session, participants spent 10 minutes discussing a particular health or spiritual issue of interest to them.

4. PRAYER (TEFELAH)

The English word prayer comes from the Greek root, precare, which means to beg (Bleck 1999, p. 288). Jews do not believe in the concept of begging. The Hebrew word to pray is l'hitpallel, which means to stand in self-judgment. Prayer has both the ability to lift human beings upward toward God and to bring God closer to human beings.

There are three types of prayers: requests, thanks, and praise. These prayers serve to sensitize the supplicants to the presence of God in daily life. Prayers are not regarded as substitutes for initiative or action. The prayers are contained within a book known as the siddur. The word *siddur* means order in Hebrew. It contains the order of the three daily services, as well as those for Sabbath and every holiday. The siddur also contains sections for special occurrences such as a full moon or even thunder.

Regardless of denomination or knowledge of Hebrew, every Jewish congregational nurse should know certain prayers that are central to all forms of Judaism. These prayers are the Shema, Mi she-Berakh, and Kaddish. Just as a stethoscope is carried by the medical–surgical nurse, so every Jewish congregational nurse should carry either a Hebrew or English version of these three prayers.

The Kaddish is a powerful prayer and well-known ritual for Jewish mourners. The Kaddish is said at least daily by family members of a deceased relative for 11 months after the death of a loved one. Although it is a prayer of mourning, it emphasizes the importance of life and does not mention death or the deceased. It expresses the hope for the ultimate healing of all people and humanity.

As noted by George Robinson in his book, *Essential Judaism* (2000), the relationship between God and human beings is not a solitary one. Mostly all the prayers (b'rahkot) are written in the first person plural. Although it is possible for a Jew to pray alone, Judaism prefers that prayer be said in a communal setting. Certain key prayers are intended to be said only in the presence of a quorum, or minyan, of 10 adult male Jews. The Kaddish is one of these types of prayers.

If a Jew is unable to pray in Hebrew, yet he or she can say Amen, this is a signal to that Jew that he or she is a part of the community (Kol Yisrael). It may happen that a Jewish congregational nurse and the client will be the only ones present to say certain prayers. Following the words of Rabbi Hillel, the nurse can safely assume that God is more interested in Jews serving other people than in serving him. In this circumstance, God can manage on his own. It is far more important for a Jewish congregational nurse to recite prayers with another Jew than not to say them due to arbitrarily dictated human requirements.

Written in Aramaic and not in Hebrew, the Kaddish is a prayer that the Jewish congregational nurse can recite with either an individual or a group of Jews receiving this type of care. The prayer begins as follows: "Yitbarakh v'yishtabah v'yipa ar v'yitromam v'yitnasie, v'yit Hadar B'yitt'aleh v'hit hala sh'mei d'kudsha b'rikh hu...."

This prayer in effect asks God for lasting peace for all peoples and their leaders in the world, as well as grace, kindness, compassion, and love for them and us. God is asked to save us from danger and distress. Amen.

CASE STUDY: THE KADDISH AND THE JEWISH CONGREGATIONAL NURSE

I was asked to visit a congregant who was reported by his wife to have a wound in his lower left leg. Athough serving as a Jewish congregational nurse at the time, I also was able to draw upon my experience as a clinical nurse practitioner. I entered the apartment, which seemed neglected. The wife told me that her husband's left leg had been swollen for some time and that he had suddenly developed an open wound on that leg. She had difficulty describing her husband's health history, so I listened intently to gather complete, accurate information. After a half hour, I realized that her husband was nowhere in sight.

I asked the wife where her husband was. She got up from her chair and pointed to the locked bedroom door. I went over to the locked door, knocked loudly, and said, "Sir, I am the Jewish congregational nurse. Your wife has asked me to come by to look at your leg wound." A few minutes went by, then a few more went by, and no response was heard. Again, I said that I was the Jewish congregational nurse and I had come to help him with his wound. Still no response. After more than 15 minutes had passed, I said to the congregant, who remained locked in his bedroom, "Sir, I need to leave now because you are choosing not to speak to me. Therefore, I cannot help you."

I stepped back from the door and slowly began to gather my nursing bag. I told the man's wife that I was going to leave shortly. I decided to ask his wife one more time about what was bothering this man so much that he refused to respond to my request to see him. His wife paused for a few minutes and then said, "Well, you know, it is his mother's Yahrzeit [anniversary of her death] and it is the first time that he has not been physically able to go to synagogue and say the Kaddish in her memory."

I decided to try once again to reach this man. I knocked on the locked bedroom door and said, "Sir, I understand that today is your mother's Yahrzeit. Perhaps if you come out, you and I could say Kaddish together." All of a sudden, I could hear the lock being turned. A few minutes passed and then I was face to face with this man. He looked as though he had not shaven in days. "Yes, I would like to say Kaddish with you in memory of my mother. Afterward, you can look at my leg."

I pulled out the prayer book from my nursing bag and we said Kaddish together. It only took a few minutes, but what a difference it made for this man. Having finished saying the Kaddish, he looked at me and said, "Now, nurse, you can look at my leg."

5. HEALTH (BREE'OOT)

Jewish ideas about health abound in both ancient and contemporary texts. Being healthy is a goal of every Jew. Perhaps no person in the Jewish religion exemplifies the importance of health in the everyday life of a Jew and its relationship with God as does Maimonides. Maimonides's full name was Moses Ben Maimon. The Hebrew acronym of Rabbi Moses ben Maimon is Rambam.

Maimonides was born in Spain in the twelfth century. He and his family fled to Morroco, later to Israel, and then to Egypt in order to avoid persecution. When his brother, a wealthy jewelry merchant, perished in the Indian Ocean along with the family fortune, the Rambam began to study and practice medicine in order to earn a living.

Also known as the greatest Jewish medieval theologian, he devoted the last two decades of his life to medical writing and practice. He became the chief physician to the famous Sultan Saladin and his family. During his lifetime, he was regarded as the leading medical authority in the Islamic world. He is widely considered by medical historians to be one of the developers of modern Western medicine. The writings of Maimonides so influenced me that the idea of health (Bree'oot) in the MJCN is based upon his writings and philosophy.

His writings contain thoughts about health, health providers, and the integration of health, religion, and spirituality. His writings state, "He shall set his heart making his body perfect and strong so that his soul will be upright to know the Lord," and "To study medicine is among the greatest acts of worship" (Maimonides 1949, p. 145).

Maimonides wrote about the sacredness of health in his code, the Mishnah Torah. Disease, he wrote, seriously diminished the human ability to achieve the highest level of spirituality. Everything that a person does in life should be directed at improving the person's physical health and the health of those around the person.

Therefore, it is an essential goal for a Jewish congregational nurse to become familiar with the writings of Maimonides so that the recipient of this type of nursing care will benefit from the nurse's working knowledge of his teachings. Although written in the twelfth century, his medical writings are as current as any found in the medical literature today.

6. VISITING THE SICK (BIKUR CHOLIM)

Visiting the sick is as old a concept as the Torah itself. The first mention of visiting the sick is in Genesis 12:13 "when God through his messengers visited Abraham after his circumcision."

Maimonides wrote down specific instructions on how, where, and when to visit the sick. "All are in duty to visit the sick. Even a man of prominence must visit a less important person. The ill should be visited many times a day" (Maimonides 1949, p. 85).

Because visiting the sick (Bikur Cholim) is such an essential part of Judaism, it is vitally important for the Jewish congregational nurse to do so, whether at the hospital, nursing home, or home setting. Establishing a Bikur Cholim board will result in allowing other interested Jews to visit the sick as well. Since visiting the sick does not come naturally to anyone, including health professionals, it will be beneficial to establish a required course for anyone who plans to visit. Practically speaking, one Jewish congregational nurse will not be able to visit all the sick who need visiting. A little help goes a long way in this regard.

SUMMARY

The Model of Jewish Congregational Nursing, with its foundations in Jewish history, philosophy, and theology has been presented so that both Jewish and non-Jewish people can appreciate the meaning of this type of faith nursing. To have a successful practice in a synagogue or community setting, a Jewish congregational nurse needs to have readily available both ancient and contemporary Jewish texts, as well as the writings of Rev. Granger Westberg. Merging these two different types of knowledge makes both the development and practice of this model possible.

REFERENCES AND RESOURCES

All online references and resources were current September 30, 2008.

REFERENCES

Abrams, J. Z., and D. L. Freeman. 1999. *Illness and health in the Jewish tradition.* Philadelphia: Jewish Publication Society.

American Nurses Association and Health Ministries Association. 2005. *Faith community nursing: Scope and standards of practice.* Silver Spring, MD: Nursesbooks.org.

Baltsan, Hayim. 1992. *Webster's new world Hebrew dictionary.* New York: MacMillan.

Bleck, Rabbi B. 1999. *The complete idiot's guide to understanding Judaism.* New York: Alpha Books.

Feldman, D. M. 1986. *Health and medicine in the Jewish tradition.* New York: Crossroads.

Ganzfield, Rabbi S. 1961. *Code of Jewish law.* Trans. H. E. Godin. New York: Hebrew Publishing Company.

Kee, H. C., et al. 1992. *Cambridge companion to the Bible.* New York: Cambridge University Press.

Lamm, N. 1998. *The Shema.* Philadelphia: Jewish Publication Society.

Maimonides. 1949. *Code of Maimonides.* New Haven: Yale University Press.

Praglin, L. J. 1999. The Jewish healing tradition in historical perspective. *Reconstructionist* 63 (2): 6–15, **www.therra.org/Reconstructionist/Spring1999.pdf#page=6**

Preuss, J. 1993. *Biblical and Talmudic medicine.* Trans. F. Rosner. Northvale, NJ: Jason Aronson.

Robinson G. 2000. *Essential Judaism.* New York: Pocket Books.

Rosner, F. 1997. *The medical legacy of Moses Maimonides.* Hoboken, NJ: KTAV.

Steinsaltz, Rabbi A. 2000. *A guide to Jewish prayer.* New York: Schoken Books.

SUGGESTED RESOURCES

To date, such resources remain few and far between, as most of the literature is at best anecdotal.

www.huc.edu/Kalsman.org   Organization concerned with Jewish spiritual and healing concerns.

www. ncjh.org   National Center for Jewish Healing

CHAPTER 9

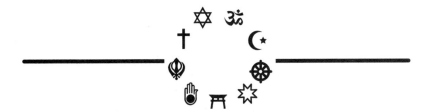

TRENDS AND ISSUES

FAITH COMMUNITY NURSES have many reasons to celebrate their specialty and all it has achieved since its beginnings in the 1980s: several thousand practitioners in the United States and the beginnings of faith community nursing in several other countries, written standards of practice, and a basic core curriculum. It took the vision and work of Rev. Granger Westberg and many others to arrive at this point. As you read this chapter, think about the issues you want to be involved in to contribute to the continuing development of this specialty.

NURSING EDUCATION

Faith community nursing leaders generally agree that a baccalaureate degree in nursing should be required for faith community nursing. This is based on the standards of practice and the responsibilities expected of the FCN. However, until there is consensus on this nationally, FCNs will continue to represent all current avenues of professional nursing preparation. It is each FCN's responsibility to practice only at his or her level of competency.

FAITH COMMUNITY NURSING EDUCATION

Developed through the International Parish Nurse Resource Center (IPNRC), a core curriculum is available to academic institutions to prepare nurses for faith community nursing. The IPNRC curriculum is one of many FCN curricula and courses available from various organizations. Work continues to update this curriculum regularly to reflect current practice. Computer technology is now being used to provide this education on-line to nurses who are unable to access other programs. The challenge is not only providing quality faith community nursing education that is affordable and accessible but assuring that every faith community nurse has the requisite knowledge and skill to practice competently.

PROFESSIONAL NURSING ORGANIZATIONS

The Faith Community Nursing Standards were developed through the combined efforts of nursing's professional membership organization, the American Nurses Association, and members of the Health Ministries Association, the professional membership organization for faith community nurses. These organizations also work to influence policy that promotes the welfare of nurses and their patients. Membership in both organizations is a professional expectation for faith community nurses.

Jackie Herzlinger, FCN, is active in the New Jersey State Nurses Association (NJSNA). In 2002 she helped form a Parish Nursing Forum within the NJSNA and, in 2005, a network of nurse leaders who are coordinators of Faith Community Programs and who are forum members. In addition to promoting and supporting faith community nursing, one of the purposes of these groups is to politically advocate for more wholistic health care services.

SPECIALTY CERTIFICATION

Faith community nursing's scope of practice has been defined and its standards of practice and professional performance described. Faith community nursing education programs prepare FCNs to practice according to these standards. Developing a national faith community nursing certification is the next logical step for this specialty. Certification provides a standard measurement of faith community nursing competence to the profession and the public. Before a certification can be developed and administered, a consensus is needed on the professional activities and knowledge areas of faith community nursing Once that is obtained, a group of faith community nursing experts can work together to develop and validate the certification, usually a several-year process that requires a substantial financial commitment. Currently a work group is exploring the portfolio process for FCN certification. A portfolio, which is the cumulative, selective record of a professional's accomplishments, is a relatively new approach to professional evaluation (Monsen 2005).

FROM PARISH TO FAITH COMMUNITY

With the recent revision of the faith community nursing standards comes the new title of Faith Community Nurse (FCN). The original title, *parish nurse,* was given by Rev. Granger Westberg, a Lutheran chaplain. Because the word *parish* was not common to all faith groups, some gave other titles to their nurses. Faith community nurse is a more inclusive title that includes nurses from all faith traditions. Even so, faith communities are encouraged to use a title for their nurse that is the most descriptive and acceptable to them. However, the specialty will be known as faith community nursing.

REIMBURSEMENT

Most FCNs work as unpaid professionals. While it is acknowledged that many faith communities would not be receiving the benefits of faith community nurses if they waited until they could afford to pay one, it is the expectation that professional nurses be paid for the work they do. Each faith community with an FCN on staff should be working toward reimbursing their nurse. The quality of each practice and the specialty as a whole will benefit from this professional recognition.

Suggestions were given in chapter 3 on finding funding to start faith community nursing programs. Because most grant funding is given to help get new ventures off the ground, faith community nursing programs usually receive such funds only as they first get started. For example, Jackie Herzlinger, FCN, got faith community nursing started in three Jewish congregations (orthodox, reform, and conservative) in the town of Springfield, New Jersey. Each congregation contributes $4,500 per year and, together with minimal grant funding, a collaborative Jewish congregational nursing program has taken shape. Jackie reports that continuing to fund this program is challenging.

LIABILITY AND INSURANCE

Liability continues to be an issue for faith communities hiring an FCN and a concern for the FCN. Faith communities and insurance companies are unsure about the liability of faith community nursing practice. The FCN working only for the faith community needs his or her own liability coverage. The FCN employed through a healthcare institution has some coverage provided by the institution. Opinions vary on whether personal liability coverage is also needed. Because opinions differ on liability, each FCN and faith community should consult their insurance carrier or get legal advice about liability insurance coverage.

DOCUMENTATION

Nursing standards require FCNs to document all aspects of their practice. To further standardize and advance faith community nursing practice, a standardized documentation form and language should be used. Work continues on standardized nursing languages such as nursing diagnoses (NANDA), the Omaha System, Nursing Interventions Classification (NIC), and Nursing Outcomes Classification (NOC). But only if nurses put these systems into practice will nursing and its specialties advance and receive full professional recognition. Until these systems are made available to nurses as computer software (and all nurse have computers accessible to them), the use and application of these systems will be uneven. It is up to each FCN to establish a form of documentation that is easily accessed and communicates nursing actions accurately and efficiently while protecting the privacy of each recipient of FCN care.

OUTCOMES IDENTIFICATION

Those in business, industry, health care, and most recently, health promotion and disease prevention programs are now expected to identify and document their results or outcomes. Ways to do this are being developed which will enable FCNs to track their interventions and associated results.

Regulatory bodies and grant foundations want health promotion programs to provide documentation and quantify the results of their services. They are less satisfied with knowing just the numbers (number of services provided, number of people reached, and levels of consumer satisfaction). Today they want to know the worth of sustained behaviors and their related consequences that can be attributed to specific services. This is a particular challenge for most health promotion programs, which have more success stories to tell than statistical data. However, methods are being developed which assign numbers to these predominantly descriptive results.

Several faith community nursing programs are considering using the outcome-based accountability system developed by Barry Kibel (1999) called Journey Mapping. Kibel's organization works with a program to document links between services provided and resulting outcomes. While financially feasible only for large organizations, aspects of the system are applicable to faith community nursing. Health promotion programs such as faith community nursing help people take steps in various change-of-behavior processes, such as losing weight or stopping smoking. Because these changes occur over long periods of time, these types of programs do not show results quickly. In Journey Mapping, results are demonstrated by identifying the links between services and outcomes and describing outcomes through telling program *stories*. Telling stories is especially useful in communicating faith community nursing outcomes.

Faith community nursing outcomes can be written up in the form of a short description. These brief reports often yield large benefits. When I included outcomes this way in my annual report, people commented more on this descriptive information than on the basic statistical reporting (such as number of people counseled, number of health classes taught, number of blood pressures taken). People said these brief stories of care were easy to read

Sample Outcome Descriptions

- A 73-year-old woman reports her symptoms to the FCN who refers the person immediately to her physician. The physician confirms the nurse's suspicion: blood clot in the leg.
- A 30-year-old male reads the article the FCN puts in the faith community's newsletter about stomach ulcers. He sees his doctor, tests positive for the bacteria, and the ulcer is healed with medication.
- A middle-aged male attends a program on cancer which the FCN offers. The FCN assesses a suspicious facial lesion. Acting on her advice, the man sees a physician, who removes a malignant lesion.
- A 73-year-old tells the FCN that "I keep running out of insulin." The person appears to have overdosed. The FCN calls the doctor. Home health care is started.

and helped them to finally understand what faith community nursing was about. Stories make faith community nursing come alive for readers.

Nursing researchers, such as the University of Iowa Nursing Outcomes Classification (NOC) group, also continue to develop outcome measurement tools. Each of NOC's outcomes, such as Spiritual Well-Being (categorized as a list of behaviors), can be used to track and measure health promotion results (Moorhead, Johnson, and Maas 2003).

Although numbers are important markers of accomplishment, Carol Hamilton, who worked as an FCN in a community center in a low socioeconomic area, makes this comment about numbers:

> I truly learned how important it is to constantly keep close to the Lord. It would have been very, very easy to fall into the trap of seeing the faith community nursing program and our own presence as valuable only in what we did or accomplished in the measurable sense. The numbers were very important in terms of getting ongoing grant support. As in all of life, the *numbers* are important, but the program will only truly make a difference if those numbers really represent God's presence in the *people* of the numbers. Right now I'm helping create more simple documentation that will hopefully keep the numbers and reporting behind the scenes for the FCNs so they can concentrate on people.

Work to make your practice measurable and accountable, communicating your results in ways that best meet your program's needs. But keep the focus on the people and the process. The health journey is just as important as the final destination.

RESEARCH

Research is needed to show the outcomes of faith community nursing as well as to develop its knowledge base. Research studies will be led by nurses with graduate degrees and assisted by those faith community nurses interested in promoting their specialty. All nurses, whatever their educational background, need to support research efforts and use relevant research results for an evidence-based practice.

FAITH COMMUNITY NURSING FOR ALL FAITH COMMUNITIES

Faith community nursing was the idea of a Lutheran chaplain, and the first parish nurses were sponsored by a Lutheran hospital. Since then, faith community nursing has spread to mostly Christian faith communities. However, there is increasing involvement of Jewish nurses practicing in their own faith communities, as well as nurses working in Muslim and other faith communities.

Just as nursing care is universal in nature, so is faith community nursing. The type of care provided will be shaped by the health needs and belief system of each faith community. As nurses of different faiths learn about faith community nursing, they will be the ones to introduce the idea to their own faith communities. This is how Jackie Herzlinger, FCN, introduced faith community nursing to several Jewish synagogues in New Jersey. She was working in hospice care when several Catholic friends invited her to a meeting of FCNs. This is how Jackie recalls that meeting:

> It hit me so hard that this concept is *so* Jewish, but Jews aren't doing it. Jews believe you are supposed to take care of your community. I saw that Jewish people were indeed taking care of their elders, but there was no *community* concept. My goal became to make faith community nursing Jewish.

Also in New Jersey, Karen Frank works full time as a congregational nurse for five synagogues in the MetroWest region. Wendy Bocarsky is founder and chair of the Reform Jewish Nurses Network, a three-year-old Los Angeles-based group that tries to bring together nursing and Jewish text skills (*New Jersey Jewish News* 2005).

As the need for community health care increases, so will the need for faith community nursing. The other countries with the largest number of FCNs are Canada and Australia. The Canadian Association for Parish Nursing Ministry (CAPNM) holds an annual meeting and has established core competencies and standards of practice. The Australian Faith Community Nurses Association (AFCNA) held its first national conference in 2005. The International Parish Nurse Resource Center (IPNRC) has established a World Forum for Parish Nursing which meets in conjunction with the annual Westberg Symposium in St. Louis, Missouri. Faith community nurses, coordinators, educators, and others interested in the global development of faith community nursing are welcome to attend meetings. Working groups have been formed to promote the growth and development of faith community nursing. For further information see the IPNRC Web site.

SUMMARY

It is exciting and challenging to be a part of developing a new nursing specialty. Not everything goes smoothly in this process. There are often disagreements and frustration. But if all faith community nurses work to make wholistic health a reality by implementing their practice standards, a common ground and unity of purpose will prevail. There are many issues yet to work on to make faith community nursing the quality practice we all aspire to. The journey has just begun!

REFERENCES AND RESOURCES

All online references and resources were current September 30, 2008.

REFERENCES

Kibel, B. 1999. *Success stories as hard data: An introduction to results mapping.* New York: Springer.

Monsen, R.B., ed. 2005. *Genetics nursing portfolios: A new model for credentialing.* Silver Spring: Nursesbooks.org of the American Nurses Association and International Society of Nurses in Genetics.

Moorhead, S., M. Johnson, and M. Maas, eds. 2003. *Nursing outcomes classification,* 3rd ed. St. Louis, MO: Mosby.

New Jersey Jewish News. 2005. A caring community.
www.njjewishnews.com/njjn.com/010506/njcaring

SUGGESTED RESOURCES

Brewer, E., C. Achilles, J. Fuhriman, and C. Hollingsworth. 2001. *Finding funding: Grantwriting from start to finish, including project management and Internet use,* 4th ed. Newbury Park, CA: Corwin Press.

Brudenell, I. 2003. Parish nursing: Nurturing body, mind, spirit, and community. *Public Health Nursing* 20 (2): 85–94.

Burkhart, L., and P. Kellen. 1999. Proposed diagnoses and interventions. In A. Solari-Twadell and M. McDermott, eds., *Parish nursing: Promoting whole person health within faith communities,* pp. 257–67. Thousand Oaks, CA: Sage.

Docterman, J., and H. Grace, eds. 2001. *Current issues in nursing,* 6th ed. St. Louis: C.V. Mosby.

Gillis, A. 1995. Exploring nursing outcomes for health promotion. *Nursing Forum* 30 (2): 5–12.

Gitlin, L., and K. Lyons. 2003. *Successful grant writing: Strategies for health and human service,* 2nd ed. New York: Springer.

Gordon, M. 1998. Nursing nomenclature and classification system development. *Online Journal of Issues in Nursing* (September 30). Available at
www.nursingworld.org/MainMenuCategories/ANAMarketplace/ANAPeriodicals/OJIN/TableofContents/Vol31998/Vol3No21998/NomenclatureandClassification.aspx

Hall, M., and S. Howlett. 2003. *Getting funded: The complete guide to writing grant proposals,* 4th ed. Portland, OR: Portland State University.

Johnson, B., P. Ludwig-Beymer, and W. Micek. 1999. Documenting the practice. In A. Solari-Twadell and M. McDermott, eds., *Parish nursing: Promoting whole person health within faith communities,* pp. 233–45. Thousand Oaks, CA: Sage.

Kenner, C., and M. Walden. 2001. *Grant writing tips for nurses and other health professionals.* Washington, DC: American Nurses Publishing.

King, M. 2004. Review of research about parish nursing practice. *Online Brazilian Journal of Nursing* 3 (1). **www.uff.br/nepae/objn301king.htm.**

Lorig, K., A. Stewart, P. Ritter, V. Gonzalez, D. Laurent, and J. Lynch. 1996. *Outcome measures for health education and other health care interventions.* Thousand Oaks, CA: Sage.

Magilvy, J., and N. Brown. 1997. Parish nursing: Advancing practice nursing model for healthier communities. *Advances in Nursing Practice Quarterly* 2 (4): 67–72.

Rydholm, L. 1997. Patient-focused care in parish nursing. *Holistic Nursing Practice* 11 (3): 47–60.

Scherb, C. 2002. Outcomes research: Making a difference in practice. *Outcomes Management* 6 (1): 22–26.

Shelly, J., ed. 2002. *Nursing in the church.* Madison, WI: Nurses Christian Fellowship.

United Way of America. (1996). *Measuring program outcomes: A practical approach.* Sales Service America.

ORGANIZATIONAL RESOURCES

Australian Faith Community Nurses Association, Web site: **www.afcna.org.au**

Canadian Association for Parish Nursing Ministry (CAPNM): **www.capnm.ca**
The CAPNM Board has developed Practice Standards and a guide for Core Competencies for Basic Parish Nurse Preparation. These documents are available at the above Web site.

Information about *Health Ministry Journal*, a publication of the Health Ministries Association, can be found at: **www.healthministryjournal.com**

The International Parish Nurse Resource Center *eNotes* is a free e-newsletter.
To subscribe:
Send a message to: IPNRC@eden.edu.
In the subject line write *Join e-mail list.*
In the body of the e-mail send your complete name, name of your faith community or healthcare organization, and your e-mail address.

The International Parish Nurse Resource Center's World Forum for Parish Nursing.
To join the World Forum, go to the Resource page in the IPNRC Web site and click on the Yahoo button on the bottom of the page: **www.parishnurses.org**

New Zealand Faith Community Nurses Association: **www.faithnursing.co.nz.**

The Pacific Institute for Research and Evaluation, Chapel Hill Center, focuses on innovative evaluation activities involving the application of the Internet-based Journey Mapping tool. Journey Mapping helps programs focus on transformation and growth processes to support their planning, quality assurance, and accountability activities. **www.pire.org/resultsmapping**

APPENDIX A

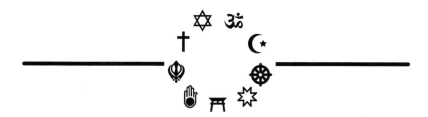

SPIRITUAL ASSESSMENT FORM

WHILE MUCH OF SPIRITUAL ASSESSMENT will be a gathering of observational data as you work with individuals and groups in the faith community, specific spiritual assessment tools and questionnaires can help in this part of FCN work by providing an explicit context for addressing specific spiritual concerns and needs. Although you may never do a formal spiritual assessment when someone comes to you with a health concern, you'll want to be aware of the ways this concern impacts their spiritual health or whether a spiritual problem might be the basis for the health problem.

Because body, mind, and spirit are constantly interacting, an FCN must consider all aspects of care. When working with people, keep these questions in mind:

- How does this physical or psychological problem affect this person's spirit?
- How does this spiritual crisis affect this person's body or mind?
- Are any spiritual concerns related to this illness?
- Are spiritual concerns the possible origin of this physical or mental illness?

And as ever: The FCN must always be sure to protect the confidentiality and privacy of any and all health or spiritual information provided by a member of the faith community.

Spiritual Assessment Form

Name _____

Age _____

Date_____

Present Concern

_____

_____

_____

Faith (Beliefs and practices)

What is your understanding of God (use term appropriate to faith community)?

_____

_____

Describe how you've experienced the spiritual dimension in your life

_____

_____

_____

How often do you attend worship services? _____

Describe your prayer life

_____

_____

Are you a member of the faith community? _____

What are your sources of strength? (*hope*)

_____

_____

Who provides help when you need it? (*social support*)

_____

What do you do when you have hurt someone or someone has hurt you?
(*forgiveness and guilt*)

_____

_____

What do you live for? (*meaning and purpose in life*)

_____

_____

Tell me what your current situation/concern/problem means to you

_____

_____

_____

Summary Statement (FCN)

_____

_____

_____

_____

_____

Signed (FCN)_____Date_____

APPENDIX B

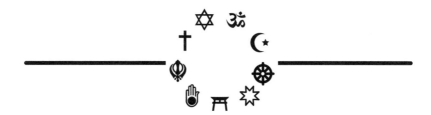

BRIEF HEALTH ASSESSMENT FORM

You can collect health information from individuals by having them fill out a health assessment form or by interviewing them. You can create your own assessment form or use a standard guide such as Gordon's Functional Health Patterns (G. Gordon 2002; *Manual of nursing diagnosis*. St. Louis: C.V. Mosby). Based my FCN learning experiences, I created and have used this Brief Health Assessment Form.

Whatever means you use, you need to be able to collect health data systematically. Taking a full health history the first time you see someone is usually not necessary, nor is it always practical. As an FCN, the only time I obtained a comprehensive history at one time was when individuals started a weight management program I'd developed, a program that included individual health counseling. Otherwise, I gathered information over time as I saw people either in my office, in their homes, or at various faith community activities.

And as ever: The FCN must always be sure to protect the confidentiality and privacy of any and all health or spiritual information provided by a member of the faith community.

BRIEF HEALTH ASSESSMENT FORM

In areas of concern, it is expected that a more thorough history will be taken.

Name _____

Date_____

Address _____

_____

Phone _____

Email _____

Marital/partner status _____

Name of physician _____

Occupation _____

Education level _____

Present concern

_____

_____

List recent changes in life

_____

_____

Describe current physical health

_____

_____

Describe current emotional/mental health

_____

_____

Describe current spiritual health

_____

_____

Religious background

_____

List medication, including over-the-counter and herbal supplements

_____

_____

_____

Recent immunizations

_____

_____

Last physical exam _____
Last dental exam _____
Last eye exam _____
Last hearing exam _____
Last mammogram _____
Last pap smear _____
Last prostate exam _____
Last colonoscopy exam _____
Present weight _____
Recent weight loss/gain _____
Present height _____

Physical limitations

_____

_____

Special diet

_____

_____

Allergies

_____

Driving limitations

_____

Smoking history

_____

Drinking history

_____

Drugs/substance abuse history

_____

Operations/surgery

_____

_____

Energy level

_____

Exercise pattern

_____

_____

Leisure activities

_____

_____

Sleep (number of hours in 24 hour period) _____

List family members/ages

_____

_____

_____

Family ethnic/cultural background _____

Family health concerns

_____

_____

Appendix B · Brief Health Assessment Form

Friends

_____

_____

Health insurance

_____

Is there anything else you want to tell me?

_____

_____

_____

_____

_____

_____

Summary Statement

_____

_____

_____

_____

_____

_____

Signed (FCN)_____Date_____

INDEX

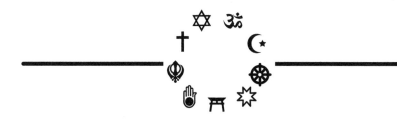